PARENTS PRAISE
DR. JILL LEKOVIC'S METHOD

"We used Dr. Lekovic's method with our two boys (three years and seventeen months) and found it to be an extremely healthy way to raise a healthy, independent, and confident child. Both of our children have enjoyed their potty time and wearing big-boy underwear since nine months of age."

—Sarah M.

"We listened to everyone who told us to wait to train our first son until he started talking. We had to struggle for months just to get him to sit down on the potty. When Dr. Lekovic recommended that we let our second child sit on the potty at a much younger age, we assumed that she would not want to have anything to do with it. We were completely wrong! We put her on the potty when she was eleven months old and she loved it. It was not long before she went to get her potty book to let us know it was time. Our potty training experience was so much happier, better, and easier, I wish we could do it all over again!"

—Michael and Lisa C.

"I had such a big conflict with my mother, who wanted to put my son on the potty before he even turned one. My pediatrician and all of my friends told me to wait, so I listened. When I met Dr. Lekovic, I learned that my son's refusal to sit on the potty after he turned two could have been avoided by introducing him to the potty at an earlier time. I followed her advice and got him out of Pull-Ups right away. Once we made going potty part of our routine, and I let him feel his own signals, his training was all over in a matter of days."

—Katharine M.

"When Dr. Lekovic told us to sit our daughter on the potty before her bath in the evening when she was only nine months old, we weren't sure what to expect. But we went ahead and got the potty, and she loved to sit on it from day one. I was completely amazed at how often she went, and so happy to know that she wasn't going potty in the bathtub every night! It really did start off an easy and natural toilet training process for us, and all of our friends thought it was amazing when our eighteen-month-old said "poo poo" and went over to the potty. We did the same routine with our son and had the same great experience."

—Brian and Stephanie S.

"It seemed like common sense to us that keeping kids in disposable diapers beyond infancy interferes with their ability to be toilet trained. So we were open to Dr. Lekovic's methods and introduced both of our daughters to the potty around their first birthdays, and got started using cotton training pants after that. We have had no problems toilet training either of our kids, and certainly never put a two-year-old in disposable diapers. Dr. Lekovic has helped and supported us all along, and we feel so lucky to have had such great advice."

—Derrick and Mara H.

"We followed Dr. Lekovic's advice with our daughter, and our photo album is filled with adorable images of our little baby happily sitting on her potty reading a book. It has been a great experience, with great results, and everyone that we know wishes that their pediatrician had given them all of the information we got about toilet training!"

—Ivan and Maria N.

"We met Dr. Lekovic after our first son was potty trained. We told her that it had been a tough process, that he started using the toilet after he turned two, and it was a daily battle just to get him to cooperate. We followed her advice with our second child, and both the process *and* the results were completely different. It was honestly a fun, sometimes challenging, but never negative, process."

—Francisco and Leah G.

"Getting our kids out of diapers earlier gave them so much confidence in so many situations, that we really believe it enhanced their development. Now when I see a parent changing a diaper on a three-year-old child, it just looks strange to me, and I am so grateful that I never did that with my kids."

—Mike and Jennifer R.

"We have listened to Dr. Lekovic's advice about potty training, and it has been such a great experience. No one can believe how well our girls did with the whole process, and we can't imagine doing it any other way."

—Peter and Salma M.

"Dr. Lekovic's plan for potty training fit with everything that we wanted for our children: to develop an awareness of their own strengths and abilities as they emerge. Watching and helping them master toilet training in such a natural way was a great experience for our whole family."

—Gena K.

THE HEALTHIER

WAY TO TOILET TRAIN

AND HELP YOUR

CHILD OUT OF DIAPERS

SOONER

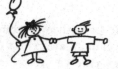

JILL M. LEKOVIC, M.D.

diaper-
free

B
E
F
O
R
E

3

THREE RIVERS PRESS • NEW YORK

Library of Congress Cataloging-in-Publication Data

Lekovic, Jill M.
    Diaper-free before 3 : the healthier way to toilet train and help your child
    out of diapers sooner / Jill M. Lekovic—1st ed.
    Includes bibliographical references.
    1. Toilet training. 2. Children—Care. 3. Children—Health and hygiene.
    4. Child rearing. I. Title: Diaper-free before three. II. Title.
    RJ61.L4856   2006
    649'.62—dc22   2005022350

ISBN-13: 978-0-307-23709-5
ISBN-10: 0-307-23709-5

Printed in the United States of America

DESIGN BY ELINA D. NUDELMAN

12

First Edition

This book is dedicated in loving memory to Dr. Punisa M. Lekovic. I sought his approval and love, and whenever I got it, held it like a treasure.

contents

Contents

acknowledgments

I would like to thank my literary agent, Jodie Rhodes, who made this project a reality. Katie McHugh, my editor at Three Rivers Press, brought clarity and focus to the manuscript. She was instrumental in increasing the accessibility of the message and the usefulness of this book. I am grateful for her professionalism, personal kindness, and many important contributions to this entire project.

The faculty of the University of Illinois at Chicago Department of Pediatrics were my first mentors. I grow more appreciative and aware of my excellent training with every passing year. I would also like to thank my parents, George and Judith Smith, for their support of everything that I do. Most important, they taught me that family love is unconditional and unchanging. My personal experience with that particular and amazing characteristic of family life made me want to be a pediatrician. The families that I work with affirm that love as an ideal for me every day. Additionally, my sisters, Jennifer Rogers and Sarah Schultz, have been the best friends and the best mothers I could hope to learn from.

My husband, Gregory, was my first research assistant, editor, critic, and proofreader. Most of all, he encouraged my passion for this project even though it meant we spent more time talking about potty training than can possibly be healthy for any marriage. I am grateful for all of his intelligence, patience, love, and superhuman optimism.

Finally, I have to thank my children, Punisa, Luka, and Eva. They are certainly the best things that I have ever been a part of, and each of their unique development inspires, teaches, and thrills me every day.

how to use this book

Diaper-Free Before 3 advocates a positive, early start to toilet training, ideally beginning between ages six months to a year, so that your child can be successfully trained and out of diapers as early as before his second birthday. Yes, you read that right—it can be done. If your child is already older than twelve months, this book will help you train your child and eliminate the need for diaper products well before the start of preschool. However, it's important to note that you can use the training method no matter how old your child is, and the exact age of completion is not the real goal or objective. Your experience with your baby is what really matters, and that should be your focus. How should you use this book? It really depends on your level of curiosity and, of course, your child's individual needs.

The organization of the book reflects my own process. I started with Big Question #1: *When is it best to start toilet training?* I have a traditional medical background, so I took what's called an evidence-based approach. This involved looking at the available studies on toilet training—describing different ages when children began using the potty over the years—and considering their conclusions based on the size and design of the study. It was these studies that drove me to dig deeper, and to find out why, in recent years, we have changed the way we go about this task and significantly delayed the start of toilet training. Chapter 1 explains this, and the rationale for my starting early.

This led me to Big Question #2: *Is there any evidence that potty training at certain ages, or in certain manners, can in any way harm, confuse, or stress out a child?* Once again I looked into the literature, but I cast a wider net to include more broadly the world of psychology. The information that I gathered served as the foundation for my plan, and so I present a modern history of toilet training practices in Chapter 2, "Life Before Disposable Diapers" (and in some detail) for that reason. To me it is compelling and fascinating. But if at any time you're ready to jump right in and start training, you can skip ahead to Part 2, "Starting Smart: Healthy and Happy Toilet Training."

• If you want to know why my recommendations seem so different from what you may have been told by others, then dig in to Part I, because the information is all there for you right from the beginning. The background really puts the plan into perspective and will give you the knowledge and confidence to move ahead with potty training.

• If you want to begin training your child, go right to Chapter 3, "The Early-Start Plan for Toilet Training." As a parent, you may be short on free time to read and just want to know what works. This book provides that in the format of an easily accessible plan, and you should start there if that is your preference.

• If your child is already older, then you should still read through Chapter 3. Even though you may feel you "missed the boat" when you read some of the ages I mention, believe me, you haven't. Keep reading, and Chapter 4, "Starting Later," offers some tips (and encouragement) on how to modify the plan if you are starting later.

• If your child has special needs, turn to Chapter 5, "Toilet Training Children with Special Needs." Again, I think you will want to read through the whole of Part 2 in order to understand the methods that I advocate, but this chapter will help you make the modifications necessary to fit your child. Most important, your child does not need to be verbal to be potty trained, and this method is ideally suited (and highly effective) for children with all types of developmental delay, including autism and mental retardation.

• If you're concerned about wetting accidents, then go to Chapter 6, "Bed-Wetting and Accidents." This issue is addressed directly there, and you will get some specific advice. Accidents are discussed throughout the book, so if you want a detailed understanding about why and how frequently accidents happen, then go back to the beginning and read more.

• If you have specific questions or are short on time, check out Chapter 9, "Frequently Asked Questions." You may find yours are discussed there. Many people prefer the Q&A format. I hope you will be intrigued enough by my answers that you will read the whole book.

There are anecdotes throughout this book, some from my experiences in training and practice, and some from my personal experiences as a mother, aunt, sister, and daughter. Some are comical (as is often the case when kids are involved), while others serve to illustrate why I feel so strongly about this topic. Whenever I mention a specific case, please don't worry about whether your child happens to fit the profile. Every child is an individual, with a personality that includes particular strengths, weaknesses, fears, likes, and dislikes, and all of these things come into play in her developmental trajectory when it comes to toilet training. Even people who have devoted their lives to this topic sometimes have a difficult time differentiating a normal child who is merely a late bloomer in certain areas of development from a child with a developmental disability or other medical problem.

You must look at your child (and each of your individual children) as a unique case. The framework of the early-start plan works for all kids, but the moment that they move from one stage to another, the number of setbacks and types of problems they may encounter will be different. Remember that the child who is toilet trained at eighteen months of age and never has an accident, and the child who still wets his bed once a week at five years of age, are both likely to be completely normal. There is nothing to suggest any difference in temperament or intelligence between the two. Your goal is simply to provide the right opportunities and encouragement at the right time to nurture your baby's natural curiosity, ability, and desire to master the potty. You can do it!

introduction

How did I become so interested in toilet training? Like many passions, mine grew out of my personal experiences. My first son was born the year I finished my pediatrics residency, and I quickly learned how much I didn't know about raising children. When you are young and inexperienced, it is easy to believe that there is one right answer to every question about child-rearing, and I turned to the many lists of reliable guidelines that are issued by the American Academy of Pediatrics (AAP). I am incredibly proud of my AAP training and everything it entailed. But as most people know, the bridge between book smarts and practical ability can be crossed only with the passage of time and the perspective of experience. That fact became apparent to me when I faced my own newborn, a tougher test of my abilities than any I had undertaken before.

My Story

I had no particular interest in potty training during my residency. In fact I never contemplated that it could be a topic of fresh controversy. Much of my pediatrics training took place at a large American inner-city hospital with patients from many countries and socioeconomic backgrounds. We learned about unique parenting customs practiced all over Europe, Asia, Africa, Latin America, the Caribbean, India, and more, all from stories shared by parents and grandparents, aunts and uncles. Many of these customs were fascinating. I heard very often about how children elsewhere were potty trained at much younger ages than we were recommending, but I attributed these stories to fault of memory (after all, who really remembers when her forty-year-old child last wet his bed?) and exaggeration. When I saw a family with their toddler in underwear, I thought it was because they could not afford diapers. I remember many physicians telling me that it was not possible to really potty train (I did not question what "really" trained meant until much later) children before two years of age, and I accepted that as fact.

Often there was a conflict apparent at an office visit between a grandmother who was trying to potty train the baby and the mother who wanted to do it the "new" or the "American" way. The mother of the baby would roll her eyes at the baby's grandmother, and tell her that with her method of early potty training it was the parents who were trained, not the baby.

Faced with these situations, I referred to the American Academy of Pediatrics guidelines regarding toilet training. These guidelines reflect what has been called a child-centered approach, most famously advocated by Dr. T. Berry Brazelton in 1962. The basic idea behind this method is that children show various signs (related to their overall development) when they are ready to be trained. Proponents of the child-centered approach argue that failure to wait for these signs to emerge before initiating toilet training can cause stress and lead to problems with accidents and toileting refusal at later stages.

Because of this background, I expected that potty training would not emerge for me as a parenting task until my son was walking and talking. But fate (or luck, depending on how you look at it) changed the course of things when he was about six months old. My husband's family came from Serbia, and we hired someone from the old country to care for our son when I returned to work. She was unbelievably good with me when I felt the pangs of new motherhood and those painful first separations from my baby, and I loved and trusted her completely.

When she wanted to start sitting my son on the potty at six months old, I said no and my husband and I had a good laugh at her "crazy" ideas. But she was so patient and persistent, and loved us all so much and so well, that we finally agreed to let her try to sit him on the little potty chair when he was almost nine months old. The rule was this: She could try to sit him on the potty once a day for a story as long as he was enjoying it. At the time, I didn't expect him to sit on that little potty at all, much less to enjoy it, and I expected her to forget about it very quickly.

But I was wrong. In fact he was so happy and satisfied sitting on that little chair, and the results were so amazing, that soon we were all hooked. My partners at work told me that I was going to regret it, that early training led to later resistance and refusal. So I decided to read everything I could get my hands on about toilet training—and there turned out to be a lot. Information about toilet training practices has been recorded since antiquity, documenting variations with regard to initiation of toilet training, methods, and outcome. The changing trends reflect the thinking of many great minds from the ancient world to the Enlightenment, the behaviorists to the psychoanalysts, the modern pediatric forefathers Sears, Spock, and Brazelton to the writings of Maria Montessori. Additionally, many experts have published studies comparing toilet training methods in different Western and non-Western countries that shed light on this issue in a broader and extremely fascinating context. (To read the findings, see Chapter 2.)

In the end I felt adequately informed to continue to train my son at his young age. Between eighteen and twenty-four months old, he was reliably dry in underwear in all settings (including birthday parties!). Yet the goal was never to train him as early as possible, but to do it in a pleasant, natural, and loving way that would feed and fuel his innate desires and abilities. He was never frustrated, and it was much easier to deal with a wet eighteen-month-old who occasionally needed a quick change into some dry pants than it is to help a three-year-old who is mad and frustrated and embarrassed about an accident that all of his playmates have noticed. We went on to train my second son with the same approach and same results, and that probably would have been the end of it were it not for two separate ongoing processes that influenced my desire to write it all down.

Why I Wrote This Book

The first of these factors was my colleagues' reactions to my personal experiences and newly acquired broad knowledge on the topic. It became a well-deserved running joke that I was obsessed with potty training, and I became a sounding board for everyone's potty training experiences. I was amazed at the number of wonderful, experienced pediatricians who would dismiss any suggestion that earlier introduction of the potty is effective, and short-circuit any discussion about the topic. I routinely received comments from colleagues that included: "You can't train a child before he is ready"; "The children will resent you"; "They will regress later and wet the bed"; and "At that age, the adults are trained, not the child." These same comments persist and are repeated with such predictable regularity that it is almost impossible to believe that they are all well established (many, many times over) in the medical literature to be completely false.

The second factor that contributed to my desire to write this book is the increasing delay in age of toilet training, the many problems this has created for both caregivers and children, and the medical problems that are on the rise as a result. The average age of training in this country is more than three years of age, and recent studies show a continued trend toward increasing delay. It is now common practice for parents to wait for their children to ask them before they introduce the potty at all (despite the fact that this practice goes well beyond even Brazelton's liberal recommendations). This is in sharp contrast to the fact that in all that is written about toilet training throughout history, up until the 1950s in this country potty training was generally completed in the first two years of life.

Today parents find that not only are they and their children frustrated, but also many preschools refuse to take children in diapers at all. The problems have been personified for me in the faces of all the discouraged mothers and fathers in the office with their three-year-old children who are ready to start preschool, able to hang from monkey bars, sing the alphabet, tie their shoes, and even copy shapes, but are still in diapers and show no interest in using the toilet. This is a bizarrely incongruous developmental situation. Clearly these children are able to be trained, but parents have been taught to fear pushing the issue. Many have not even purchased a potty for the child, as he does not "seem interested." Most are not even aware that their situation represents a radical departure from basic and centuries-old child-rearing practice that has potentially serious consequences.

The Potty Myth

Where did we get the idea that troublesome lifelong issues involving every aspect of personality development, overall adjustment, and even sexuality can develop from toilet training a child too early? I try to answer this question in Part 1 of this book, but suffice it to say that even though many experts have tried for years to establish some such connection, this myth has not been remotely established in any way. After a thorough review of the medical and psychological literature I can state without reservation that there is nothing inherently psychologically stressful about toilet training, and I establish this in the coming chapters in detail. Moving from diapers into independent toileting, as a developmental task, is analogous to moving from a diet of exclusively milk to self-feeding solids. These processes both require intensive caregiver involvement, but no one would suggest that the introduction of baby cereal is likely to harm the baby psychologically, even if she doesn't particularly like it at first.

All parents know that times of stress, illness, or fatigue can cause disruptions not only in potty training but also in a child's diet, sleep, and general behavior patterns. This fact underscores the importance of good parenting in general, of a predictable routine and a secure and loving environment for all children all of the time, and does not suggest special psychological significance associated with toilet training. Deciding to avoid toilet training because children sometimes have accidents when they are tired or distressed makes no more sense than, say, avoiding introduction of solid foods because months or even years later that child may cry for a bottle when a new baby is brought into the house.

Over-Reliance on Disposable Diapers

There is one anecdote that sticks out in my mind as an example of the misinformation parents routinely receive about toilet training. It involves a family that had adopted a fifteen-month-old baby from overseas. The adoptive parents came to their (caring and experienced) pediatrician when they returned to the States. They reported that they had seen the baby cooperating happily with the potty in the orphanage and, after many extended visits with the baby, had never seen him wet or soil his pants. They questioned the pediatrician about how to handle this situation now that they were back with the baby in suburban America. He advised them to put the baby back in diapers until he was able to tell them that he needed to go, which is what the parents did. This baby had a reliable potty routine and had not wet himself for months! It is impossible to predict how this individual baby would have done with toilet training in the middle of all of the adjustments of an international adoption, but there was absolutely no reason not to give him the opportunity of keeping that routine and building on it.

The disposable diaper industry has an enormous interest in keeping the "delayed training is better" message prominently reinforced, and encouraging parents to use their products for longer and longer periods of time. Many diaper manufacturers have incorporated into their advertising campaigns the suggestion that it is better for the child to be trained later. In fact disposable diapers are readily available at any supermarket in larger sizes than could be purchased only one generation earlier. I remember writing prescriptions less than a decade ago for disposable diapers for children weighing more than thirty-five pounds, because they were considered medical supplies for children with disabilities. Today the majority of children wear disposable diapers or Pull-Ups well beyond this size. The cost to parents and profits to diaper manufacturers and advertisers involved in keeping children in diapers an extra year (and beyond) is enormous. There are specialists in medical journals regularly suggesting that this trend has negative health consequences, but no voice within the profession has spoken out. It is clear that using highly absorbent materials to diaper our children for ever-longer periods of time has altered the process of toilet training, but no one has directly addressed what those effects might turn out to be.

The Benefits of Starting Early

• *The sooner you start, the sooner you finish.* Studies show that the age of starting training clearly affects the age of completion. When parents are told not to begin too early, then kids aren't successfully trained until later ages. Many older children resist and even refuse toilet training. Depending on when you begin, you can have your child using the potty around his first birthday and completely out of diapers as early as his second.

• *Kids learn their natural signals faster.* Prolonged use of disposable diapers causes children to be trained at much later ages by limiting or eliminating the natural signals of wet and uncomfortable. Most parents of a newborn baby know that she is fussy when she is wet or dirty. The fact that parents frequently report that their toddler "prefers" to have a bowel movement in her diaper suggests a troublesome alteration in a basic set of instincts.

• *Easier socialization.* Mastery of toileting skills provides children with confidence and abilities that enrich many areas of their development. A number of preschool teachers have commented to me about the difference between a three-year-old in diapers and one who is using the potty. Once he is out of diapers he is no longer a "baby," who needs to be changed by an adult, and he (and his peers) sees himself as much more independent. He is more aware of the abilities and functions of his own body, and even able to plan on appropriate times to go potty. These abilities give him an amazing amount of confidence in the (often frightening) world of preschool socialization. It is also much more hygienic to have children using the toilet than it is to have groups of children together in diapers.

• *Some children never show an independent interest in training.* There are some parents out there waiting for the right moment when their child seems interested, and eventually their child is four years old and no one knows what to do because the child seems perfectly happy to continue to use the diaper. You can avoid this by introducing the potty in babyhood.

• *Decreased risk of urinary tract infections and accidents.* Several medical problems have emerged that are linked with delayed training. The development of bladder control involves a complex set of physiologic processes involving not only the muscles of the bladder but also many intricately linked events in the nervous system. Urology experts have expressed concern that delayed training has led to increased rates of voiding disorders and lasting wetting problems across the population. Urologists argue that the delays in training suggest a fundamental shift away from actually training children to empty their bladders at regular intervals (which is how children have been trained throughout history), and toward teaching them to await a sense of urgency before making the trip.

• *Decreased risk of constipation.* Increasing rates of constipation among children have led experts to suggest possible cause-and-effect relationships with potty training. One is that children are constipated more because they are not being potty trained properly from a young age, so they are holding their stool too long (because they don't want to go in the diaper, or don't want to take the time to go to the potty) and becoming constipated as a result. The longer that they try to wait and avoid a bowel movement, the harder it gets, and the more that it will hurt. You can prevent this cycle by training your child not to refrain from having a bowel movement by making sitting on the potty a part of his routine.

Reaching Success

I believe that parents should measure the successfulness of their toilet training by looking at the whole child's happiness and adjustment over extended periods of time. Staying positive goes a long way toward more contented mealtimes, easier toilet training, and happier family life in general. I have seen too many parents spend a great deal of time postponing or avoiding potty introduction because they have been told there is something wrong with even approaching this topic with their child. By the time they get around to it, they are often faced with a toddler (or preschooler) who is too busy doing other things, and too attached to her sense of autonomy, to have anything to do with the brand-new potty that suddenly appears in her environment and seems to disrupt her day.

The combination of this evidence has shaped me into a bona fide potty training evangelist, and I've tapped into an unexpected personal wellspring of enthusiasm for it. In the end it's clear to me that teaching and encouraging children to use the potty from a young age is not fundamentally different from all of the other things that we help them to do. The goal of *Diaper-Free Before 3* is to avoid unnecessary stress, help your child stay healthy, and make potty training a happy, shared bonding experience between you and your child. Reintroducing yourself to the process can teach you many amazing things about your baby and, at the very least, will give you a lifetime of memories.

modern potty training

HOW WE GOT HERE
AND WHY IT MATTERS

P
A
R
T

what's wrong with the idea of readiness?

The parents of a healthy one-year-old boy, Jake, bring him in for his regular checkup. His growth is normal and his parents report that he started taking a few steps on his own over the last few weeks. He says "mommy" and "daddy," shakes his head no and yes, and looks around for his shoes or favorite toys when they are mentioned. He was weaned from the breast two months ago and now only takes a bottle before bed and nap. He loves a variety of foods and does well drinking from a cup.

Jake wears disposable diapers, and his parents have noticed that his diaper is often dry after a nap and that his bowel movements are usually after breakfast and dinner. He is curious about the toilet and wants to go in with his parents. He loves to have his diaper off and even tries to take it off himself at times. Jake's pa-

ternal grandmother got him a little potty chair for his first birthday, and his parents have a lot of concerns about when to introduce it. Their friends have told them that it is "way too early to even think about it." They want to know how to tell if he is ready to be toilet trained, and how to avoid making any mistakes along the way.

Is Jake ready to be toilet trained? Most doctors and parenting books recommend that children must show signs of readiness before beginning toilet training. Different experts list various skills, but most suggest that children require some communication skills, a desire to use the potty, and the ability to walk to the potty before being trained. Before you decide when it is best to start training your child, you should know that these guidelines (and the very idea of readiness) are based on the well-publicized *opinions* of a few individuals (not medical research), and are by no means infallible.

When you look at the history of potty training, how it was done in the past and under different circumstances, and how we came to consider the readiness guidelines to be the standard, you will begin to question what you have been told and to seriously reconsider what is best for your child. Despite the fact that a review published in the May 1999 issue of *Pediatric Annals* stated that "there is little question that children can be toilet trained by one year of age," most parents (and doctors) are not even aware that there is a well-established alternative to toilet training based on readiness skills.

Over the last century, changes in American lifestyles

have been complex and far-reaching. Many of the changes in the perception of children and the practice of child-rearing are closely linked with these more general trends in our society. The most influential development with regard to toilet training was the introduction of Dr. T. Berry Brazelton's child-centered approach to training, a concept that has led to the current American Academy of Pediatrics (AAP) guidelines for toilet training. In this chapter I will explain the current guidelines and how they evolved. I will also explain how this approach is based on a false set of assumptions and theories (many of which have subsequently been established in the medical community to be mistaken). The readiness approach may actually pose multiple health risks to your child, inadvertently impeding her natural course of development.

The American Academy of Pediatrics Guidelines for Toilet Training

The idea behind child-centered training is that children show various signs (related to their overall development) when they are ready to be trained. The AAP lists several signs of readiness, including:

- *The ability to walk to the potty*

- *The ability to understand and follow one- and two-step commands*

- *Adequate language skills to express needs and wishes*

- *The child's desire for independent control of bowel and bladder function*

The guidelines suggest that once you see these signs of readiness in your child you should gradually introduce your child to the potty. Most people see these signs begin to emerge during the second year of life, and the usual time to start training based on these guidelines is around two years of age. However, observing development is very subjective, and many children do not have much useful vocabulary in the second year of life. Many people see verbal communication skills (or a lack thereof) as an obstacle to potty training their child based on these guidelines, and they put off training because they do not know how to train a child who can't (or won't) tell them when he needs to go. Furthermore, the child's desire for control must be recognized by the caregiver and can mean anything (depending on the parent's interpretation) from pulling off the diaper to wandering into the bathroom to actually asking to use the potty. That means a child could seem ready at twelve months, or not until he is three years old, just based on how much he talks (a skill that has nothing to do with actually using the toilet), or on how curious he seems to be about the toilet. A lot of this has to do with the parent's expectations, and if she does not think a child can be trained at fifteen months of age, she will not think her child's curiosity about the potty has anything to do with toileting readiness.

Although these guidelines are well intentioned, they are based on some faulty assumptions and have led to some huge delays in toilet training and unforeseen consequences. The average age for completion of training has advanced from before eighteen months (in the 1970s) to thirty-six months and beyond. The AAP guidelines are completely open to interpretation and have not provided adequate guidance to help parents understand their children's development. There has been a shift in what we recognize in our children's behavior and abilities, leading to even further delays in training. There are no instructions about the use of disposable diapers or suggestions about when it might be appropriate to stop using them. There are also no comments about accidents, how many to expect or consider normal, or how to handle them. Finally, the idea that it is potentially harmful to your child to introduce the potty before he is ready is neither based on any medical facts nor supported by the many studies that have been done on this topic.

Dr. T. Berry Brazelton

The guidelines used by the AAP developed (to a large degree) from the work of Dr. T. Berry Brazelton. Dr. Brazelton's approach centers on the signs of readiness from the child, such as communication skills to express needs and motor skills to be independent with the task. He advised mothers to gradually introduce their infants to the potty after eighteen months of age, which at the time of his study was a huge delay for most people. He urged parents to avoid using pressure, in order to facilitate the infant's independent control of toileting. He argued that bowel control at age two or three was strictly a developmental task (or something that a child will "grow into"), as opposed to a skill that needed to be taught or practiced.

These recommendations evolved from Brazelton's famous 1962 article called "A Child-Oriented Approach to

Toilet Training." In the introduction to this article he states: "Since the advent of streamlined diaper care has liberated mothers in our culture from the real need to 'train' their children early, this step may be viewed more honestly as a major developmental task for the child." I realize that I am looking at this from a different point of view, but who says women needed to be "liberated" from caring for their children? Furthermore, how could the invention of disposable diapers made of paper and plastic materials that were created in the last few decades (after human beings have been dealing with this issue for thousands of years) allow us to *finally* see the task more "honestly"? It simply does not make sense. It was the same (patriarchal) medical establishment that convinced an entire generation of women that giving their babies formula saved them from the onerous, time-consuming, and unseemly task of breast-feeding. Since then, it has become evident that there are many health benefits to breast-feeding (not to mention some mothers who think it is a wonderful, important experience to share with their babies).

Brazelton relied heavily on psychoanalytic theory to make the case that delaying toilet training was not only more convenient but also desirable from a developmental standpoint. He argued that children trained at a younger age were more prone to regression under pressure (or having accidents), and that this could be avoided by confronting this task at a more advanced stage of development. Writes Brazelton:

> Parents and pediatricians are aware that the child's autonomous achievement in any developmental area frees

> him to progress to more advanced areas. Faulty mastery
> may leave him with a deficit that results in regression
> under stress. [Pathological symptoms such as constipation
> and enuresis] . . . usually reflect a fundamental psycholog-
> ical disturbance in the child's adjustment.

In short he felt that there was a connection between problems with potty training and the child's psychological well-
being. This was not a new idea (I discuss a little history in
Chapter 2), but Brazelton popularized it in a way that
changed how everyone viewed toilet training. He took toilet training from being a natural part of a child's growth
development and made it one with special psychological
significance.

Myth #1: Toilet Training Has Special Importance in Children's Psychological Development

Many experts have questioned the connection between
toilet training and psychological disturbance in children
over the years. Even one of the most popular and well-
regarded pediatric reference textbooks, Nelson's, states:
"There is little to indicate that the experiences involved in
the toilet training of most children are of major psychological consequence." Of course being negative, humiliating,
or punishing a child as a part of toilet training can damage
her self-esteem and cause her to resist training. But these
patterns reflect an underlying parental approach and atti-
tude that impacts all areas of child development, not just

toilet training. You should use the same measure of patience, flexibility, and love with toilet training that you do with all of parenting.

Myth #2: Babies Don't Know When They Are Voiding

Since Brazelton did his 1962 study, we have increased knowledge about the developing nervous system in babies and children. As part of his argument for later training, Brazelton referred to theories suggesting that babies are born with a simple reflex occurring at the level of the nerves in the spinal cord, which causes them to empty their bladder when it is full. The idea was that as the bladder fills, certain nerves sense it is full and those nerves directly set off a corresponding set of nerves that lead to the bladder being emptied. According to Brazelton's theory, voluntary control of voiding happens only when the brain matures enough to begin to control this simple reflex. This is clearly not the case, as the current medical evidence proves.

Today's experts have found that newborn babies already have brain-based control over voiding related to arousal. In fact PET scans have shown that specific areas of the brain become active in newborn babies before they empty their bladders. This means that the higher functions of the brain are getting some sensory input and then exerting control over the bladder in a way that is much more complex than a spinal reflex arc, even before birth. There are certain stages in the sleep cycle when the bladder does not empty. This fascinating area is wide open to research, but it is clear that Brazelton's assertions do not explain the system. The idea that there is a transition at some point in the child's development from reflex voiding to voluntary voiding, or any point when higher functions of the nervous system are *not* involved in voiding, has been completely discredited. So these facts shift the question from being "When does a baby's brain become involved in voiding?" to "When does a baby become consciously aware of these processes?"

This question of conscious awareness in babies presents itself in many forms. Parents often see their newborn baby smile, and many have asked me when babies know they are smiling or begin to smile on purpose. Usually I give a simplistic explanation that there are many expressions that occur spontaneously in babies, but they begin to recognize and smile at caregivers after about six weeks of age. The real answer is a little more complicated, but analogous to toilet training.

Facial expressions in babies can represent spontaneous events, or they can be responses to stimuli as simple as the discomfort of being cold or having gas or as complex as a feeling of comfort, fear, or even happiness. The differences among when your baby is unconsciously moving his facial muscles, when he is responding to his environment with reflexive grimaces and smiles, when he is imitating the expression of a caregiver, and when he is making the connection among seeing a caregiver, feeling happy, and deciding to smile about it are not measurable, at least with what is currently known about the cognitive development of humans. They occur over time and not at a single moment.

Bladder and bowel control are similar things in that there is a gap between what is possible in terms of conditioned behavior and when babies become aware of the process in the complex sense that involves anticipation, planning, and communication. This complex but completely apparent fact directly confronts the idea that the signs of readiness suggested by the Academy have real significance. As much as we wonder as parents what our babies think and feel when they smile, we accept that we really don't know, and we continue to smile and talk to them as they grow. The same should be true with potty training. There is no specific age when children become aware (or for that matter any age when we know that they are *not* aware) of their toileting needs. We should offer them cues to tune in to the signals from their bodies (see your baby flushed and grunting, take him to the potty, he feels relaxed sitting on the potty, and he has a bowel movement).

Myth #3: Early Training Causes More Frequent Accidents

This assertion has been completely disproven many times over since it was first made. In fact there is no evidence that children trained early have any increase in the amount or frequency of accidents throughout childhood. The opposite is true; children trained earlier have much more reliable and consistent control than older children who often make accidents one of their tools in their ongoing power struggle with caregivers. Most children go through episodes of increased frequency of accidents after they have been trained, and there does not seem to be any association between training method and these periods.

Brazelton advanced the theory that the ability to be voluntarily trained (and thus to be able to control accidents) correlated with development of certain parts of the central nervous system that control voluntary motor functions. He argued that this process occurs between twelve and eighteen months of age, and any training prior to that time would lead a child to regress when she entered later stages of development.

But a lot has changed in our understanding of the nervous system since the 1960s, and these innovations must be applied to Brazelton's arguments about the neurological development of children. It turns out that there is no point at which it can be argued that a nerve starts working, and no evidence that taught behaviors at any age could interfere with the development of the nervous system. Instead the voluntary activity of the nerves that control the muscles involved in toilet training develops in the same way as all areas of physical development in childhood, starting in the embryo and becoming continually more coordinated and controlled throughout childhood in a relatively predictable fashion.

If Brazelton's assertions about the development of the nervous system are flawed and outdated, why are parents still being taught these toilet training guidelines? The development of each child is an individual and variable process.

The Myth of Readiness

Brazelton also advocated the idea that there is a "transfer of developmental energy" from one task to another; that is, a child can learn only one new thing at a time. He claimed: "The developmental energy invested in learning to walk on his own is freed after 15 to 18 months and can be transferred to the more complex mastery of sphincter control and training." However, the current understanding of child development directly contradicts this notion. Neurological development occurs as a predictable and co-ordinated series of events. A child's abilities to walk and to be independent with toileting occur at about the same time because she is influenced by some of the same factors with regard to physical development. There is no such thing as the "transfer" of developmental energy from one task to another. In fact there is no such thing as "developmental energy."

An individual child's development is influenced by a complex sequence of neurological processes that is in turn influenced by genetics and, to some very poorly understood degree, by the child's environment. Although the child's habits and behaviors can be modified, her physical maturation appears to be unchanging.

The truth is that there is no physical or developmental marker of toilet training readiness in children, and no point when it has been established that there is some benefit to delay training. Many experts have looked into this issue in increasingly complex ways, always concluding that the marker of readiness that they were considering was either frequently absent in children who were well trained or frequently present in children who weren't. These suggested markers have included the size and function of the bladder, the maturation of the nervous system and brain, and the development of language skills and cognitive abilities. In many cases the ages at which these systems mature from an anatomic or physiologic standpoint are known to be much later than would correspond with any suggested age of toilet training.

For example, a group of researchers did a study looking at the maturation of the position of the bladder neck in children. This feature of physiologic development was thought to correlate with the ability to control urination. While the researchers did find that the position of the bladder neck changes from infancy into a mature or adult position, there was no connection between when that happened and toilet training. In fact many children in their study were fully trained (and continent) years before their bladder neck was in a mature position.

In effect the parent's expectations of successful toilet training have a lot more to do with when a child is trained than do any markers of development. This does not suggest, of course, that the child does not have a central role in the process. Toilet training, like all aspects of parenting, should be responsive and sensitive to the child's needs and abilities. An approach that is truly centered around the child involves recognizing her capability, desire for mastery, and frustration with diapers long before the readiness guidelines would suggest they are present. For a two-year-old child, there is a huge difference between the pride and comfort associated with a bowel movement on the toilet compared with the frustration and discomfort associated with having a dirty diaper and needing to wait to be wiped clean and diapered by a caregiver.

It doesn't make sense to define the child-centered approach as one that waits, effectively, for the child to train himself. A two-year-old child may lack the verbal skills to tell parents he wants to go potty but have an entirely predictable routine that would keep him clean most of the time and allow him the satisfaction of using the potty that provides the foundation for complete potty independence. Furthermore, children between two and three years of age are very prone to develop a power struggle over the potty if it is thrust upon them during this window. If they are already familiar and have had some experience with success with the potty, many will see it as an opportunity for increased autonomy to really master the task. Parents often tell me about their twelve- to twenty-four-month-old babies "going crazy" during diaper changes, trying to escape, screaming, and trying to arch their backs or squirm away. As we pin them down and wipe their bottoms off, maybe we should consider the idea that this is their sign of potty training readiness.

Just like other areas of childhood development, toilet training involves a process of early imitation and learning, followed by the gradual understanding of more sophisticated patterns, and this progression is important to recognize. By comparison, during the development of speech, a child first imitates sounds that she hears in her environment. Later she begins to respond to her parents' verbal cues ("Say dada") and then imitates actual words based on positive reinforcement from caregivers. This basic pattern of conditioned response is gradually replaced by increasingly sophisticated use of language as the child matures. Between two and three years old her vocabulary explodes, and she has the foundation to develop more complex communication skills as she develops increasing intelligence.

There is no connection suggested between the early response of a caregiver to a baby's babbles and his ability years later to form sentences. No one suggests that rigid parenting might harm the neurological development of language centers in the brain (although severe neglect or abuse can cause language delay). By direct comparison the connection between the early introduction of toilet training in a loving environment and later regression seems absurd.

Babies acquire language skills from their environment based on their own pattern of cognitive development. If a mother cooing "Mama loves you" to her baby every night before bed leads to that baby eventually saying "Mama," we see the beauty of learning in babies resulting from the routine, daily loving care for them. Their toileting skills should come in the same way—from observation, exposure, opportunity, and practice, with lots of pleasant interaction and positive reinforcement from caregivers.

Why Early Training Makes Sense

For Children's Development

The child's nature is to aim directly and energetically at functional independence. Development takes the form of a drive toward an ever-greater independence. It is like an arrow released from the bow, which flies straight, swift and

47

sure.... While he is developing, he perfects himself and overcomes every obstacle that he finds in his path.

—Maria Montessori, THE ABSORBENT MIND

Children have a natural drive and desire for mastery and independence. As part of their developmental process, most will begin to imitate adults as soon as they are able. Everyone has seen small babies pretend to talk on the phone, demand to grasp the real keys, hold on to pens and pencils, grab the remote control, and scream to have the fork or spoon someone is eating with. This is not because these objects are by nature fascinating, but because they are the things they observe the adults around them using all the time. They want to master their environment and be allowed to develop the ability to do their daily tasks independently. Toilet training is central to this self-mastery, and for that reason it is important to start early and give them increasing control over the process. The first step in this process is getting them out of diapers so that they can experience what is happening with their bodies, giving them a potty, and teaching them how to use it.

Most parents are not even aware that in most parts of the world, and in this country one or two generations ago, children would have been independently using the toilet long before we are now even introducing it. (I will discuss this more in the next chapter.) Caring for a twelve- to eighteen-month-old involves almost constant caregiver attention, and this relationship is ideally suited to introduce toilet training. A two-and-a-half-year-old or three-year-old has developed a strong desire for independence and a natural desire to say no when told what to do, no matter how attractive the parents try to make it seem. There is no evidence to suggest that children successfully trained at an early age are likely to regress or go back to having frequent accidents in the later toddler years. In fact data (and experience) show that the average two- to three-year-old prefers to already be independently using the potty and takes great pride in her mastery of this task. Furthermore, there is emerging evidence that suggests that the prolonged use of disposable diapers can have lifelong consequences to the function of the urinary system. (I will discuss these developments in Chapter 7.)

Rather than child centered, I think the readiness approach is adult centered, if the convenience offered by disposable diapers amid our increasingly hectic lives has led most people to avoid this admittedly inconvenient but important project of toilet training. The adverse effects of later training have clearly emerged as older children often show increased resistance to the initiation of training. Pediatricians like me are faced daily with wonderful parents who have dutifully followed all of the AAP's recommendations about introducing the potty based on their child's signs of readiness, but their child is showing no interest and continues to demand a diaper. Parents commonly express concerns that they will create a stressful conflict with their child if they encourage her to use the toilet. However, many studies have shown this to be untrue.

For Socialization

Delays in training lead to delayed socialization, as many children are not allowed in preschool environments if they are not trained. It also results in the incongruous but common observation at any park, library, mall, or playgroup of three- and four-year-old children who can run, climb a ladder, swing from monkey bars, tell stories in full sentences, and even write the letters of the alphabet while wearing disposable diapers. How a given child feels about being in diapers at this age is a difficult thing to assess, as he doesn't know much beyond his own experiences, and there is a complex interplay between his desire for mastery of adult-like tasks and his natural instinct to resist relinquishing control to caregivers. But I am certain, all other things being the same, that no child would prefer to go on wearing diapers if he was properly taught and encouraged about using the toilet.

Parents are commonly utilizing complex motivational and reward systems to coax their bright and savvy toddlers to try the potty. I have heard about every imaginable treat being offered to children for going potty, from candy to stickers to performances by Mommy involving pom-poms and dancing. Doesn't all of this seem a little bit strange for such a natural and universal process? I find it impossible to imagine a Victorian or Early American mother trying to entice her son to use the potty by aiming at targets of Cheerios, or promising a certain number of pieces of candy for successful urination or bowel movement. Handling toilet training much more matter-of-factly, building it into your child's routines of mealtimes, sleep, going outdoors, and bathing from a young age, will naturally preempt the need for this type of theatrics and rewards. Children have a natural desire be capable of doing things themselves, particularly with regard to self-care, and all they need is an opportunity and some guidance. If you can ask your child to go to the changing table and get a diaper and wipes and bring them into the living room so that you can change him, then I promise you (without exception) that you can potty train him. And, more important, everyone will be happier.

To Decrease the Risk of Infectious Diarrhea and Hepatitis A

The delay in toilet training has also caused problems that are associated with group childcare. Multiple studies have shown higher rates of both infectious diarrhea and infectious hepatitis in children in diapers in group-care settings than in children of the same age who are toilet trained. Of course it is obvious why a group of preschoolers who spend a lot of time on the floor, touching many toys and other objects with their mouths, might have bacteria or viruses spread from crawling around in a full diaper or from having their hands in and around their diapers without washing them. There is also the extra spread of germs by caregivers changing multiple children's diapers.

Most two- and three-year-old children are so detail conscious and obsessed with their routines that once they are taught to wash their hands after using the potty it is next to impossible to rush them through it, much less to convince them to skip it. I find that this makes for better germ control than counting on caregivers (however good our intentions are) to take the time for a good hand-washing after every diaper change when they are constantly pulled to attend to other things.

The increased incidence of diarrheal illnesses in group-care centers with children in diapers compared with children who are toilet trained is so significant that there have been several articles by public health officials recommending earlier toilet training for all children in group care, and several vocal advocates for delayed toilet training have stated that the health benefits for children in group care may make it preferable to train those children earlier. In particular, a child is too young to be immunized against hepatitis A until she has passed her second birthday. So she is vulnerable to this common (and occasionally very serious) infection at a time when she is starting to explore and learn from her environment, often by putting everything into her mouth. Multiple studies have shown that the transmission of hepatitis A is much lower in childcare environments where children (regardless of age) are toilet trained.

For Urinary System Development

Over the last sixty years there has been an increase in cases of lower urinary tract dysfunction among children. It has been suggested for years that delayed toilet training might play a role. A report in the *British Journal of Urology* in 2002 found a strong association between the lack of formal bladder training that occurs with delayed toilet training and permanent bladder dysfunction in some children. Voiding problems lead to such problems as incontinence, urinary tract infections, and urge problems (basically a frequent need to urinate on short notice). Most of these problems have been found to occur in people who are neurologically normal, and the problems relate to the function of the bladder. Urologists call this problem nonneurogenic bladder dysfunction. This study found significantly more problems with both day and night wetting in primary school children who were trained after eighteen months of age and also when scheduled voiding was used less. In short, children who were left to go when they had the urge (in most cases holding urine in their bladder for a prolonged time), without any structure, reminders, or schedule, were more likely to develop these problems.

For Lifelong Healthy Bowel Habits and a Healthy Lifestyle

Likewise the increasing rates of constipation among both children and adults in Western countries have been a cause for concern for many years. Numerous adult medical problems have been linked to constipation, from diverticulosis to hemorrhoids to colon and breast cancer and diabetes. The discomfort and embarrassment associated with childhood constipation causes the whole family significant distress. Many experts have speculated on issues contributing to the increase in this problem, the two leading factors being diet and toilet training. The effects of diet are complex, and it is beyond the scope of this book to discuss them in detail, but I do give some general guidelines in Chapter 8.

There is a close correlation between the rising age of children being toilet trained and increased rates of constipation. This has led to the argument that the failure to teach children to have the patience and good habits necessary to sit on the toilet at appropriate times throughout the day (i.e., the failure to actively toilet train them), has led them to hold their stools (or delay having a bowel movement) much more frequently than individuals who were trained the old-fashioned way. The longer that children delay or avoid having bowel movements, the harder their stools become because the body absorbs more water from the stool the longer it sits there.

There are a lot of reasons that children avoid having bowel movements, but the most common one is that they are busy and do not want to interrupt what they are doing. If they learn to sit on the toilet at appropriate times throughout the day, these trips seem like a routine instead of an interruption and are therefore resisted much less frequently. It often doesn't work to ask a two-year-old if he would like to use the potty, not because he does not understand the question or have an ability to control the process, but rather because he does not choose to stop what he is doing to go to the bathroom. If he sits on the potty for five minutes after every meal as part of his schedule, then it starts to make sense to him to use this time to do something (like go potty). If it is established as a routine, then children lose their desire to avoid it. They develop the (quite sensible) idea expressed by my first son every time he asked us, "After we have dinner, go potty, and wash our hands, can we go outside?" It just fits into the normal sequence of life. Parents can also become more aware of their child's bowel movements and can start to understand what type of diet allows their child to have soft, regular bowel movements from a very young age.

So the idea of potty readiness developed out of some interesting theories, but these theories have not been supported by more than fifty years of medical science. The sentiments they suggest seem innocuous and even appealing (Who wouldn't want to wait for their baby to be ready to do anything?). But as with many things it turns out that a nice idea can be interpreted or used in the wrong way, or it simply may not apply to a specific situation, and such is the case with potty training readiness. Parents have been convinced that there is something inherently dangerous in training their child before she is ready, and there is simply no evidence to support that that is true. Waiting for readiness signs has caused parents to refrain from training their children until long after what has been considered normal and natural for centuries, but the benefits of earlier training are numerous. To put things into a broader context, the next chapter describes potty training practices in the past and in other cultures. Now that you understand where we are, it is time to look at how we got here—and just what people did before disposable diapers.

life before disposable diapers

The parents of a delightful eighteen-month-old girl, Sadie, come in for a checkup. She is growing well, is off the bottle, and eats a balanced diet of table foods. She uses several words (including "mama," "dada," "no," "shoes," "milk," "ball," "baby," "dog," "go," and the occasional "me, too"). She runs well, tries to help dress herself, and scribbles with a crayon. Playful and curious, Sadie loves to get a reaction from those around her. She sleeps well at night and takes a reliable afternoon nap.

Her parents report that she has two soft bowel movements most days and occasionally comes to her parents if she wants to be changed. I suggest that they start dressing her in cotton training pants during the day. Their immediate response is "Are you kidding?"

We all laugh, and I reassure them that they are not alone in their fears about starting this project and leaving behind the convenience of disposable diapers. It is a big transition, but she will love the freedom it gives her, and it will allow her to learn. After all, in the past (and of course present) parents everywhere somehow managed life without disposable diapers.

Put into the context of the history of toilet training, the idea that there is a point when children are ready to be toilet trained is really quite new. In fact it wasn't until the 1960s that it was widely accepted that children need certain skills before being toilet trained, and by that time disposable diapers were used across the population. After that point the two separate things (the idea of toilet training readiness and the use of disposable diapers) became part of one concept: that children should remain in disposable diapers until they show signs of toileting readiness. Before that children wore cloth diapers and were held over the potty beginning in the first year of life based on a routine schedule (such as after feeding or when the baby awakened), as well as when caregivers recognized various signals from the baby (such as wincing, grunting, straining, or fussiness). These early attempts to "catch" urine or stool in a potty led to traditional potty training based on the baby's schedule. Most children were reliably trained before their second birthday, well before many people today would suggest that they were ready to learn. And caregivers reported being able to tell by the baby's behavior if he needed the potty, relying on his predictable routines (such as urinating upon awakening and stooling after eating) to determine when to try.

The Convenience Factor

The first step in the toilet training process is deciding when to start. In the first part of the twentieth century, when training began in the first year of life, parents anticipated that it would be a long process with intensive involvement on their part. It makes sense that if you have a baby in cloth diapers that you have to clean, then any opportunity to have the baby use the potty instead of a diaper is considered a success and worth the effort. A baby in a cloth diaper also complains quickly when wet or soiled, and she develops a rash if not changed promptly, so there is more labor involved and more awareness of the baby's schedule and needs. Disposable diapers absorb wetness so the baby often does not even feel it, much less express any discomfort to caregivers. You can imagine that if you had to clean all of the laundry (and I don't mean load the washing machine) every time your baby used her diaper, then you would be more motivated to observe her and begin to predict when she was going to void or stool. If she became more uncomfortable, too, because she felt the wetness of the cloth around her, then you would get more clues from her about what to expect. When you consider that historically preschool-age children spent most of their time around the home, cared for by family members, with a household routine that required frequent changes of cloth diapers and an unavoidable awareness of the baby's schedule for wetting and stooling, then early potty training seems practical and convenient.

The idea that it is more difficult and time consuming to start training earlier developed after people began using modern laundry facilities, and it grew with the widespread use of disposable diapers. It became easy to deal with soiled diapers with less effort, and the motivation for investing a lot of time in toilet training diminished. Not only did it become easier to clean soiled diapers, but disposable diaper materials also made it more comfortable for babies to stay wet or dirty for prolonged periods of time, taking diaper changing from a routine of every two hours to an event happening only a few times every day.

The importance of convenience with regard to childcare in general increased as a result of social trends that emerged around the same time. As more women entered the workplace, and more families were separated by relocation, it became more common for children to be cared for in a group setting. It became part of the routine in most group-care environments to keep children in disposable diapers for longer periods of time in an effort to ease the demands on caregivers.

Even the at-home mother was increasingly spending time out of the home with her children—on the go, in the car, at various activities, and running errands. Modern conveniences may have freed women from spending the whole day cooking and cleaning at home, but everything that goes into keeping that modern life running has led to a frantic pace in our lives that leaves little opportunity for labor-intensive (and home-centered) childcare. Because no one is home to cook, we eat out or else consume premade food at home, and the detriments to our health are increasingly understood. In the same way, we have continued to delay toilet training because of the time investment required, without really understanding the consequences.

The first disposable diapers became widely available in the late 1960s. Not coincidentally the readiness, or child-centered, philosophy emerged at around the time that these social trends were gaining momentum, making it very easy for disposable diaper manufacturers to promote the idea that not only is prolonged use of their products convenient for parents, but it is preferable and beneficial to the child. I don't think there was any kind of organized conspiracy to trick people into using these products; rather all of the events in our society that brought women out of the home (including not only education and career but also the availability of personal transportation and the sprawl that resulted) happened around the same time as disposable diapers became available. Over the years these products have become increasingly sophisticated and can absorb huge amounts of liquid without leaking or even feeling wet. Most people who used those early disposable diapers in the 1970s, even through the 1980s, remember how they ballooned up with each void and would start to leak if not changed pretty quickly. Now made with modern materials (available since the late 1990s), disposable diapers are so highly absorbent that they can easily hold an entire day's worth of urine without leaking. In fact it is often hard to tell if they are even wet after a single void.

But where has this left us? All of these things have contributed to the increasing delay in toilet training, and in many cases the actual burden falls on the child who is sitting in a soggy diaper in her car seat long after she would have been toilet trained by old-fashioned methods. We have gone too far with our fears of giving up diapers. It is possible to do better by our children with toilet training without going back to the Dark Ages for women. I have seen many people (including myself) with complicated lives that include jobs, school, and personal commitments that pull them in many directions, who must often put their children in all types of childcare arrangements from in-home, to daycare centers, to shared nannies and extended family arrangements, *all* successfully (and very happily) go about an early potty training plan.

When Is a Child Successfully Trained?

Before we look at the studies on this topic, know that the definition of successful training varies by study as well as by culture and tradition. Some individuals classify a child as trained when he is able to void or stool when placed on the potty some of the time, even if the child frequently wears diapers or has accidents. Today it is common to regard children as trained only after they are able to independently use the bathroom without prompting and without accidents or bed-wetting.

This variability in the perception of the process does color these studies' conclusions. If you believe that your child is not trained until she can go to the bathroom alone without any reminders, then of course she will be trained later than if your definition allows for you to prompt her or to help her with her pants. There is not a universal definition among experts of when a child is officially potty trained, and many of these studies use arbitrary definitions such as "less than one episode of daytime wetting and two episodes of bed-wetting a week," or some variation of that. It makes it impossible to directly compare numbers in different studies if their definitions are not the same, but the general trend can be seen and understood without the benefit of more exact comparisons.

I have found this to be true in my personal experience, as well. If I ask a parent in the office "Is he potty trained?" the answer I get often says more about the parent than the child. Some people say yes, and when I ask a follow-up question like "Does he ever have accidents?" they will say "only once or twice a week." Another parent might answer no to the initial question, and then to the follow-up will say "He has accidents at least once or twice a week." If I didn't ask the second question, then one of those children is trained and the other is not, when in fact they are the same.

The Timeline

The methods and timing of toilet training have fluctuated widely over time. The changing attitudes have largely resulted from societal trends rather than medical or scientific discoveries. As I describe the timeline you will see the gradual increase in age of initiation of training over time. I often hear the suggestion that stories of early toilet training represent revisionist history on the part of individuals from either a different generation or a different culture (or both). These people suggest that older generations simply don't remember (or they exaggerate) when they trained their children. But the medical evidence states otherwise. Many, many studies have been done describing toilet training practices in this country since the late 1800s, as well as in other countries and cultures. All of them clearly show that children have historically been trained much earlier than they are today. Parents need to know the real history.

Toilet Training, 1890 to 1950

Attitudes toward children in the period between 1890 and 1910 were characterized by permissiveness and indulgence. Mothers in 1890 were chiefly interested in the development of a good moral character in their children. Child-rearing practices were designed to produce children who would exemplify "the Victorian ideals of courtesy, honesty, orderliness, industriousness and generosity; character, not personality, was the focal point."

Two separate articles published in the early 1950s analyzed popular parenting advice from 1890 to 1950, with an effort to describe the timeline of changing attitudes among American parents. The first paper, written by Dr. Celia Stendler, reviewed articles about child-rearing that appeared in popular magazines (such as *Good Housekeeping* and *Ladies' Home Journal*) between 1890 and 1948. The second paper, written by Dr. Martha Wolfenstein, analyzed a set of booklets published between 1914 and 1951 by the United States Children's Bureau entitled *Infant Care*. These booklets were widely read parenting guides and underwent several drastic revisions in those decades.

Turn-of-the-century parenting writers emphasized using

rewards (including smiling and praise) throughout toilet training. In 1914 writers advised beginning bowel training by the third month or even earlier. But important emphasis was placed on gentleness, as "scolding and punishing will serve only to frighten the child and to destroy the natural impulses, while laughter will tend to relax the muscles and to promote an easy movement." The plan was to sit the baby on the potty at the same time each day in an effort to establish bowel regularity. Most parents used a small baby pot for this purpose.

The 1920s

The 1921 revision of *Infant Care* showed evidence of increased severity, demanding training in the first month of life. Interestingly, the comments about the importance of gentleness and laughter were absent. The 1929 edition called for more rigorous bowel control, emphasizing doing everything "by the clock" to promote absolute regularity. Experts even recommended using a soap stick to stimulate the rectum to bring about the movement at the appointed time. This edition argued: "Almost any child can be trained so there are no more soiled diapers to wash after he is six to eight months old."

The trend toward greater control in training technique resulted from the rising popularity of the psychologist J. B. Watson. He was at the center of the behaviorist movement that came to dominate the field of psychology for the first half of the twentieth century, which focused on ways to describe and control behaviors. He encouraged strict adherence to a schedule in an attempt to condition the baby to have the desired behaviors. The infant was viewed as passive, and by nature any spontaneous response to a child's desires was discouraged.

In fact, though inadvisable, these types of methods actually do work from a physical standpoint. Lightly stimulating the rectum of a baby will often result in a bowel movement, and with time many people set a routine so that the baby naturally emptied his bowels at that time. The desire for control over the baby's natural processes that led to this type of practice, however, has been widely discredited and denounced. Setting up a relatively predictable routine in a baby's life where he eats, sleeps, and is changed on a regular schedule is clearly beneficial to the child. He thrives with that predictability and is comforted by the familiarity of a schedule. Physically forcing him to have a bowel movement at a certain time of day by putting something in his rectum is an entirely different matter, and much of what happened later in terms of the field of child psychology was a reaction against this type of manipulation and rigidity.

The 1930s to 1940s

With the emergence of new ideas about child development based on the advancement of psychoanalytic theory, the early 1930s brought a partial return to increased permissiveness with regard to toilet training. The notion that each child is an individual with a unique personality and set of abilities and that it could be beneficial to consider these things in raising that child is central to modern, Western child-rearing and education. The psychoanalysts placed great emphasis on how the attitudes and behavior of the caregivers early in life might affect the child's development. Early psychoanalysts advocated the predominance of nurture (or external factors) over nature (or inborn traits) in the development of a child's personality and overall adjustment. For much of the twentieth century most of the discussion about child development in general and toilet training specifically hinged on a basic acceptance of these assertions and their widespread application.

Stendler found that by the 1940s the number of women's magazine articles about personality development in the child had eclipsed all other topics. Authors frequently pointed out the importance of understanding the underlying cause of a certain behavior rather than focusing on controlling the behavior. Since nurture was now associated with the development of certain personality types, cautions against spoiling the child were replaced by the argument that problems with development were related to flawed or inadequate mothering. The psychoanalysts argued that placing excessive pressure on a child at any point could lead to faulty development, and this idea was applied very literally and broadly to toilet training.

The psychoanalysts argued that toilet training occupied a central position among several inherent psychosexual conflicts in the child, the resolution of which was formative for later personality traits. Out of this thinking developed the idea that rigorous demands placed on the child early in life could cause him to repress, rather than resolve, his innate conflicts, leading to later psychological problems. The development of a well-adjusted personality overtook the notion of good character as the goal of successful parenting. It was widely accepted that the methods used by parents in

everything from feeding to toilet training had lifelong implications in personality development. Sigmund Freud is
the most famous psychoanalyst, and most people are familiar with the associations he made among toileting habits,
sexuality, and general outlook on life.

Because of this dramatic shift in philosophy, Dr. Harold
Orlansky conducted a large review of the data on the relationship between methods of infant discipline (specifically with regard to breast-feeding versus bottle-feeding,
self-demand versus scheduled feeding, weaning, thumb-
sucking, mothering, and bowel training) and personality.
His study, published in 1949 in an article entitled "Infant
Care and Personality," concluded that there was no connection between a general parenting method and later personality development. (This is not to suggest that it does not
matter how children are treated or raised. It simply reflects
that you cannot make a direct connection between what
type of parent you are and what type of personality your
child will have.) Dr. Orlansky found no scientific basis
for the revolution in child-rearing, and he attributed the
changes to general social trends. Amazingly his conclusions
(based on a review of the experimental and anthropologi-
cal evidence) were largely ignored, and individuals in the
field continued to frequently assert a connection between
method of toilet training and personality development.

The 1950s

Dr. Benjamin Spock published the first edition of *The
Common Sense Book of Baby and Child Care* in 1946. He
argued for a return to a gradual, passive approach to toilet

training. This meant postponing training until the child was beginning to sit with stability, around the sixth month of life (obviously, still early by today's standards). This trend gained momentum throughout the 1950s with several sociological factors combining to influence modern toilet training dogma. These factors include the changing role of women in our society, the separation of families by relocation and sprawl, technological advances ranging from the widespread availability of automobiles to near-universal use of disposable diapers, and the emerging field of psychology that has changed how we view human beings and their development.

Drs. Robert R. Sears, Eleanor E. Maccoby, and Harry Levin published a report in 1957 entitled *Patterns of Child Rearing*, which resulted from a larger study undertaken by the Laboratory of Human Development of the Harvard Graduate School of Education. In it, they analyzed standardized interviews with 379 American mothers of five-year-old children to determine the factors that contributed to their child-rearing techniques. They addressed the issue of toilet training and compiled the answers to create a general picture of the approach to this task. During this time, the average age at the beginning of toilet training was eleven months, and three-quarters began the process before fourteen months of age. The average duration of training was seven months, and 90 percent of the children completed training before their second birthday.

This study is important for several reasons. First it confirms the fact that early introduction to the potty (and completion of training) was the norm even into the 1950s in this country. Second it shows that regardless of training technique there is an age *range* for successful completion. This is one of the hardest things to remember for parents who are aware of every aspect of their child's development and are so frequently exposed to comparisons with all of the other children of the same age in the family, in the neighborhood, at playgroup, and at church.

Another aspect of training that Sears addressed was the severity of pressure from the caregiver. He counted both very frequent and prolonged attempts at the potty, as well as punishment for accidents, as measures of severity. He established that severe methods did not speed up training but did add to the child's signs of resistance and emotional upset over the process. Note the important distinction between "structured" potty training and "pressured" potty training. The whole idea behind early introduction to the potty is that you make sitting on the potty a normal, positive part of your routine from an age when your child is most open to it. In most cases this will mean less conflict and pressure put on your child, as you will avoid the trappings of a power struggle that might emerge if you introduced the potty at a later age. You should encourage your child to cooperate by making the whole experience a natural part of your loving care for her at an age when her whole world revolves around her caregivers. Threats of punishment, much less actual punishment, have no role here.

The 1960s

A group of Swiss doctors conducted a study of the growth and development of a group of children between 1955 and 1976. This study was performed on a population that was still using cloth diapers and practicing old-fashioned training techniques. At three months of age the mothers held 13 percent of their children over a pot or the toilet. By six months of age this number increased to 32 percent, and by twelve months 96 percent of their children had begun on the pot. The results demonstrated that 60 percent of the children showed partial and 35 percent complete bowel control by the end of the first year of life. By two years of age three-quarters and at three years practically all of the children were completely trained to use the potty for bowel movements.

In this study bladder control was separated into control by day and by night. By two years most children had at least partial bladder control. Of interest, 20 percent of the children showed complete bladder control (no accidents) by two years of age. The third year showed 78 percent of the children were dry except for occasional accidents, increasing to 89 percent at age four and 97 percent by age six. Partial bladder control at night was established in 50 percent of the children by two years of age, meaning that they still had occasional nighttime bed-wetting. By three years of age most children were partially dry at night, with 20 percent completely dry (no bed-wetting). During the fourth year of life the majority of children became completely dry at night, and by six years old more than 90 percent had complete bladder control.

This study is important because it demonstrates the results of early potty training in terms of timing of completion and frequency of accidents. At this time the American public was converting to readiness criteria and delaying training until the second year of life. Most of the articles and recommendations coming out at that time in this country argued that starting training earlier would *not* lead to later age of completion, and this study helps clarify when children were trained without using the readiness criteria on a large population. Obviously, with the benefit of hindsight the age of initiation of training *does* affect completion, and this is demonstrated by this study.

The 1970s to 2002

Since 1970 many studies have been published that reflect advancing age of initiation of training in Western countries. Most are conducted on children in disposable diapers, cared for in their homes by their mothers. Today the average age for initiation of training has gone from around eighteen months in the 1970s to between twenty-four and thirty months. The ages of completion of training have similarly advanced from before eighteen months to thirty-six months and beyond.

In a 2002 study published in the journal *Pediatrics*, the authors reported that parents recognized their children "showing an interest in using the potty" at twenty-four to twenty-five months of age. The median age of staying dry during the day was almost three years of age for boys and girls. When you look back at Sears's 1957 study (not much time elapsed between the two studies) and consider that Dr. Sears reported that almost all of the children started training before eighteen months of age, with more than half completing the task by eighteen months of age and another quarter (so a total of 84 percent of the children) finishing before twenty-four months of age, then the sudden delay in toilet training is shocking.

The same 2002 study reported that parents recognized their child "indicating a need to go to the bathroom" between twenty-six and twenty-nine months of age. To me this is one of the most amazing statistics that I have seen. As we have noticed in study after study, from different points in history caregivers have been able to reliably pick up on cues from babies that they are going to void or stool starting in the first year of life. The majority of parents surveyed in 2002 (with children in disposable diapers and awaiting

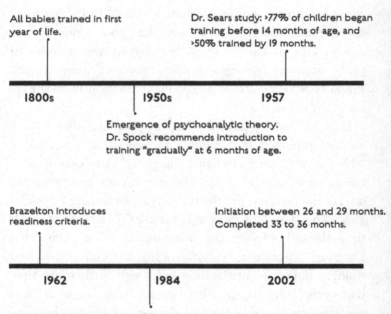

All babies trained in first year of life.

Dr. Sears study: >77% of children began training before 14 months of age, and >50% trained by 19 months.

1800s · 1950s · 1957

Emergence of psychoanalytic theory. Dr. Spock recommends introduction to training "gradually" at 6 months of age.

Brazelton introduces readiness criteria.

Initiation between 26 and 29 months. Completed 33 to 36 months.

1962 · 1984 · 2002

Stanford University study: 45% of children began training before 18 months of age, and 37% began between 18 and 24 months (82% by 24 months).

today's widely accepted readiness signs) did not notice any indication from their child until close to the third birthday. How much of that is due to the fact that the child simply isn't aware because he doesn't feel the wetness in his disposable diapers and how much of it is reflective of changes in what we recognize and accept about children's abilities is not known, but clearly kids *can* be trained by age two.

It *Does* Matter When You Start!

It is clear how the average age for starting training has increased dramatically over the last few generations. But how has this trend changed the average age of training completion? Several of the studies I mentioned previously included numbers clearly suggesting that earlier introduction leads to much sooner completion. In fact in recent years multiple other studies have looked into this question specifically, with an effort to control for other variables, and have come to the same conclusion—the sooner you start, the sooner you finish.

• An American study published in 1997 reported that when toilet training was initiated before twenty-four months of age the majority of children were trained before age three; while of the children who were introduced to training after twenty-four months of age only half were trained before age three. This study is important because it was the first to suggest an adverse effect for delayed initiation. When starting later almost half of the children were still in diapers at that critical three-year-old age mark.

• Another study published in the journal *Pediatrics* in 2003 looked at toilet training practices in a group of suburban children. The authors found a direct correlation between age of initiation and age of completion of training. The age range for completion of daytime training was twenty-two to fifty-four months (yes, that is four-and-a-half years old). It is important to note that the correlation between earlier introduction of training and earlier completion was even stronger when intensive training methods were used. They defined "intensive" training as asking the child to sit on the potty more than three times a day. That does not constitute intensive training in my opinion (or by historical standards), and I think even most modern parents think that reminding their child to go potty three times a day is not extreme. In this study there was no association found between earlier or intensive toilet training and constipation, stool withholding, or stool toileting refusal.

• A group of doctors in Japan published a paper in 1987 that found the age of initiation of toilet training is the only factor that contributes to when it is completed. Babies who began training between twelve and seventeen months of age were most likely to be independent of diapers at thirty months of age.

The one factor that strongly influenced when toilet training was begun was living with grandparents. The Japanese found that in the 1980 group, toilet training was begun at 17.6 months of age for infants who lived with their grandparents, and 68.4 percent of those children were trained by thirty months of age. Children who did not live with grandparents were begun at 20.6 months of age, and

58.4 percent were diaper-independent by thirty months of age, a highly significant statistical difference. You could argue that living with grandparents simply means there are more people available to care for the baby and invest time in toilet training, even without a big philosophical difference among generations with regard to toilet training. But that data still supports an argument that earlier introduction to the potty means earlier completion of training.

• A group of doctors at the Children's Hospital of Philadelphia published a study in 2004 to determine which factors contributed to delayed training. They looked at toilet training methods, frequency of constipation, birth of a sibling, and childcare arrangements. Their study included collecting data on the child's temperament and language development. They *also* looked at parental expectations, parent/child relationship, parental stress, isolation, attachment, health, depression, and spousal relationships. Statistical tools determined what role each of these variables had on age of toilet training.

The conclusion? The only factors that seemed to play a significant role in age of completion of training were the age of initiation of training and the presence of constipation. Children who have frequent hard or painful bowel movements tend to delay or avoid toilet training as a part of their overall desire to withhold bowel movements. It has been established in several studies that problems with constipation occur *before* problems with toilet training (and in fact in most cases *cause* the problems with training), and I discuss this topic in detail in Chapter 8. None of those other factors (including birth of a sibling and parental

The Digo Perspective

Looking at toilet training practice in a culture isolated from both Western parenting advice and Western commerce and products offers an interesting comparison. The Digo are a Bantu-speaking people living in the Indian Ocean coastal plain in East Africa. Dr. Marten W. deVries undertook a study of the toilet training habits of 110,000 Digo that was published in 1977. In this study mothers of three- to twelve-month-old infants, selected at random, were questioned about their expectations for bowel and bladder training of their infants. The majority stated that they initiated training during the first few weeks of life and expected or had accomplished reasonable night and day dryness by four to six months.

Digo mothers expected full dryness by one year of age. They accomplished this by being in almost constant physical contact with their babies. After the caregivers (either the mother of the baby or a young girl from the family) developed a sense of the baby's behavior associated with voiding (such as when the baby wakens, stirs, or complains), as well

as the baby's overall schedule with regard to eating and sleeping, they became able to tell when the baby was going to void. They would then hold the baby over their knees in a certain position to facilitate voiding. Accidents were considered the caregiver's mistake, for failure to recognize what the baby needed. The idea that the responsibility for recognizing the need to void rests with the caregivers is in sharp contrast to the responsibilities that our society places on the older child.

There is a natural comparison between the very rigid training patterns practiced in this country in the 1920s and the early training practiced by the Digo. However, it appeared to Dr. deVries that this was not the case. He argued that the Digo viewed their infants as active, not passive, participants in the process. Furthermore, their training style was based on a set of cues that both the mother and the baby learn. DeVries called this "the growing acquaintance of mother and child."

This seems to be the ultimate example of child-centered toilet training, where caregivers are ex-

divorce) were found to be associated with the age of successful toilet training in any way.

So there really was life before disposable diapers, and toilet training in much of the twentieth century was clearly a different experience. The suggestion that children need to be ready to be trained seems like one small spot on the timeline of social and cultural trends, a fad that grew out of a lot of interesting debate and discussion. It was impossible for those early advocates of delayed toilet training to predict the influence that their theories would have on people's actual toilet training practices, much less the problems these changes might cause in the whole population. We have the benefit of that information now, and we should use it. There is no evidence that waiting to potty train children benefits them in any way. In fact the continued delay in training has created problems for them that are only now being recognized and explained.

OVERVIEW OF THE PLAN

STAGE	GOALS	AGE WINDOWS*	COMPLETION
INTRODUCTION	Baby gets comfortable sitting on the potty.	Starting between six and twelve months of age, continuing until between nine and fifteen months of age	When baby regularly cooperates with sitting on the potty at least once a day
PRACTICING	Baby starts to occasionally void and stool on the potty. Pattern develops that involves multiple trips to the potty throughout the day. Baby spends increasing amounts of time in cotton underwear.	Starting between nine and fifteen months of age (whenever baby seems comfortable with more frequent trips to the potty) Completion anytime between twelve and twenty-four months of age	When baby has found a routine that keeps her clean and dry most of the time without constant supervision and reminders
GOOD HABITS	Maintain good habits that include drinking plenty of fluids, eating the right foods, and having regular bowel movements.	Between twelve months and three years of age	Lifelong

* These age windows are suggested, but if your child is already older than these ranges, know that you can immediately introduce your child to the potty and move through the stages from there. For more information on training an older child, see Chapter 4.

starting smart

HEALTHY AND HAPPY TOILET TRAINING

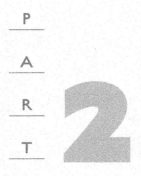

P
A
R
T

2

the early-start plan for toilet training

T
H
R
E
E

Before You Start

Before you can begin toilet training you have to get a potty. There are many styles of children's toilets out there, and I think every home with a six-month-old (or older) child in it should have one. A baby needs a few basic things in life, and one of them is a potty that fits his body. The best come with as few pieces as possible, as they feel more stable and last longer. There should be some support for the baby's back, even though he may lean forward at first. It should be a normal object in your house long before your child is particularly aware of it, and it should be sitting there in the bathroom so the first time that the thought crosses your mind that he might be able to sit on it, you can give it a try.

It has become popular for many people to skip the training potty entirely and introduce their child to the regular toilet with a little seat on top. Part of the reason for this is that people are starting training when their children are already getting too big for a little potty chair. There are several reasons why skipping the little potty is less preferable. First, it is much more difficult for the child to get onto an adult potty, and there is always the possibility of a fall. Second, many children are frightened of the water, of falling in, and of flushing. Finally (and most important), the ideal posture for both voiding and stooling involves some support for the feet. Can you imagine climbing onto a toilet that was so large that your feet could not touch the ground and then trying to have a bowel movement? You must have your feet on the ground to properly use those pelvic muscles, and so should your child. The famous developmentalist Dr. Arnold Gesell argued in 1949 that a small potty that allowed the child's bottom to be well supported with her feet on the ground was essential, and that fact remains true.

Having a little potty in the bathroom also makes it possible for you and your child to go potty together. This can be very helpful with training, even with opposite-gender parents, as she sees you go through the little routine of going to the bathroom and washing your hands, and she has such a strong desire to imitate you. I have often found myself in the uncomfortable position of going through the whole routine of getting everyone to the potty, dressed, and with shoes on before we head outside, only to realize I forgot to use the bathroom myself. This is a secondary benefit (but an important one) to having a small potty: Keep the big one available for the adults. Most children express a desire to use the regular potty by the time they are three or four years old, and of course you should support that transition when they are ready. If they want a little step stool, encourage them to use it as a footrest as well, as that will really help them use their muscles effectively.

Once you have the potty you have to think about the plan to use it. I have read in some of the old articles that people defined the beginning of training as the first time they had a child's potty in the home. I think that is a great place to start, and it makes everything else seem less dramatic (as it should be). The goal is not to train kids early as some mark of their precocity or intelligence but to give them the familiarity with the process that provides them with the opportunity and the skills to go about the task in the way that suits them. Too often by delaying training we are failing to give children who would be much happier going on the potty the chance to do so. The process of toilet training occurs over three phases that I have labeled: introduction, practice, and good habits. The idea is to focus on the process and the specific objective of the phase you are in, and to avoid the common mistakes made when expectations are not well understood.

Before you start it is important to understand a few basic things about your baby's body. Babies empty their bladders at regular intervals. Modern technology has demonstrated that this is true even before birth. At no point with a normal baby does urine simply dribble out constantly. There is a system in all babies where the bladder fills up and then at some point the signal comes to contract the muscles that empty the bladder, and this occurs every few hours. This occurs around twenty times a day in a normal newborn baby. It is important to know from the start that there is no real understanding about (and probably no specific age or time) when the baby becomes aware of this process. Instead there is a gradual process of growth and development occurring over time involving not only the growth of the baby's bladder but also increasing awareness of his body and his environment. Once you recognize how gradual this process is, and you see the great satisfaction your baby has as he begins to put the pieces together, you will find it easy to stick to the plan.

Phase 1: Introducing the Potty
(As Early As Six to Nine Months of Age)

Putting your baby on her potty for the first time should be no different from putting her in her high chair. Most parents try their baby in the high chair when they think that her trunk and neck are strong enough to be comfortable sitting. Some babies cry at first, but you make adjustments and find a way to make them feel comfortable and secure. You may try to distract them or give them something soothing or pleasant, or you might take them out and try again later. This is the same process to use for the potty.

Some babies are more open to new experiences while some react negatively to everything at first and then warm up with time. It is the same routine as with the bathtub, car seat, crib, and stroller. As you use them more frequently they become familiar objects and experiences to your baby. These transitions are particularly difficult with your first baby, when you feel that you might be doing something wrong. The truth is, every baby comes with a unique personality and you just have to figure out what works through trial and error. Your baby may like you to be exuberant and clap your hands and smile at him as you sit him on the potty, or that may terrify him and you need to find a different approach. Trust yourself, pay attention to your baby, and you will figure out pretty quickly how to make potty time just as pleasant as your feeding and bathing rituals have become by now for all of you. The most important thing to remember is that in early development, babies thrive on routine and predictability.

This first trial at the potty should ideally occur some time between six and nine months of age. When your baby is able to sit independently with some stability, but before she has really taken off and is crawling (and you are chasing her) all over the place, there is a period of time where her favorite thing is to sit across from you with you at arm's reach (or in your lap) and hear you talk or show her a book. Babies are particularly attached to caregivers at this age and it is often difficult to even walk out of the room they are in for a moment without a complaint. It is a labor-intensive stage in childcare by nature. Independent play is rare, and babies at this age enjoy and thrive on lots of attention and interaction with caregivers. They are becoming more aware of what goes on in their environment and are curious about the objects (the phone, the keys, your fork, the remote control) that they see you using. This is the moment to introduce the potty. If your child can pick up the phone, imitate how you talk on it, and devote most of her energy to trying to get whatever you have (or whatever has your attention), then she will probably love to sit on the potty just like you.

The main goal of this phase is to make the child familiar and comfortable with the potty and be able to sit there with a caregiver for at least a few minutes regardless of whether he goes. Some children at this stage like the ritual of a single familiar toy or book that they look at while sitting on the potty, and small board books are ideally suited for this purpose. Some babies require something new and interesting every time. Many babies at this age will just want you to sit there and touch them and smile, talk to them, and give them your attention. Remember, we are talking about only a few minutes, so there is no need for elaborate entertainment.

At this phase it is totally appropriate to start teaching your child the words that go with the potty, and repetition helps. Some Indian parents have told me that they make a "whoosh-whoosh" sound every time they sit the baby on the potty to help him to urinate. I think that anything that strengthens the routine and makes the whole experience more familiar will help. I usually sit on the floor right in front of my baby and say something about using the potty and then show him a board book, often while holding on to one of his hands or stroking his leg or feet.

The first few times your baby may lunge forward or act uncomfortable, but give her a chance. Try to distract her to get comfortable and give her your attention, as that is what she enjoys most of all. Many babies prefer to lean forward so that their feet can touch the ground (if they can reach) to feel comfortable. Try different positions on the seat, but concentrate on reassuring your baby that you are right there, smile and laugh, and show her something pleasant and distracting. If she does not want to sit down, just smile, get her dressed, and then try again later. Do not feel discouraged, and definitely don't feel frustrated or disappointed with your baby.

The secondary goal of this stage is becoming aware of your baby's routine, in order to know when he is most likely to cooperate, most likely to be impatient, possibly ready for a bowel movement. You use all of your knowledge and familiarity with your baby's patterns to determine when and how often to sit him on the potty at this stage. One of my children started waking with a dry diaper before he was a year old, and as long as I responded to his first round of "Mommy!" yelled from his crib in the morning and got him right to the potty, he would empty his bladder there and that was how he really took off with toilet training. Another one of my children did not wake up dry until he was almost completely potty trained (and older), and he had much more success after meals. You should not be stuck with a set of expectations, even if this is not your first child. Pay attention to what works, to when he seems cooperative and happy to go, and keep track of when you usually have success.

Childcare

You have to make your plan fit your life, so you must take into consideration practical issues such as childcare. In

Early Training in Group Childcare:
The Montessori Method

In a Montessori toddler community (which is made up of a community of toddlers from fourteen to sixteen months [walking stably] until sometime between two-and-a-half and three years), we have several approaches to help a child become independent in toileting.

First we create a physical environment with a very low toilet, a low accessible sink, and a supply of training pants (either individual or communal supply). This can be done at home with a ring on the toilet to reduce the size of the hole, a large stool in front of the toilet, a stool to the sink, training pants on a rack, and a basket on the back of the toilet.

When a child arrives, and says good-bye to Mom, we calmly aid him in getting ready to enter the working area of the community. In some places this means changing into indoor shoes. In all places it means taking off the diaper (usually paper) and donning a pair of underpants. Clothes on top of the underpants are not ideal (more challenging to get to the toilet)

but in some areas are mandated. Ideally the child wears a shirt, underpants, and indoor shoes until he is getting a handle on going to the toilet.

About an hour and a half into the morning we begin to see a change in the movement of the group—a kind of restlessness. There is more aimless moving about. At this time we simply say to one or two children (not the entire group), "Oh, it's 10:30; it's time to use the toilet." The younger child very dutifully goes off to the bathroom, sits on the very low bench, helps pull the training pants down and off, and goes to sit on the toilet. She urinates, defecates, or simply sits on the toilet for a bit (no prescribed amount of time—this is up to the child). Following this, she helps in getting dry, clean underpants on, washes her hands, and returns to her work/play. So, working with one or two children at a time, all the children are invited to use the toilet. A child can always refuse.

A similar announcement is made prior to going outside to play, before eating, and before and after napping (if the child sleeps in the community). "Oh, it's almost time to go out. First we use the toilet."

Gradually children are more and more successful. They arrive to a point where, when the adult makes the reminder announcement, they check in with their own bodily awareness and either go off to the toilet or declare they don't need to go.

Finally they reach the stage when they become aware enough of their own bodies that they no longer need a reminder. They simply go when they need to.

We don't say to a child—even if his body movements indicate a need to use the toilet—"I think you need to use the toilet."

We don't refer to wetting or defecating in the pants as "having an accident." This is what we say when we get hurt and need a Band-Aid.

We don't coerce children to use the potty. We don't reward them when they "make a deposit." We simply treat it as normal as eating, which of course it is.

There are many communities worldwide where this is the common practice; of course in many other cultures, delayed toileting is not an issue. It is the expectation that children will normally be trained between twelve and eighteen months—once they are walking.

—Judith A. Orion

Association Montessori Internationale (AMI) Director of Training The Montessori Institute, Denver, CO

Australian Montessori Teacher Education Foundation, Sydney, NSW

Montessori Laboratory of Educational and Environmental Psychology, Osaka, Japan AMI, Amsterdam

Board of Directors Pedagogical Committee Sponsoring Committee

most situations it is easiest and best for your baby to first be introduced to the potty at home and then to increasingly introduce the potty in different environments and with different people. There are numerous wonderful childcare centers that practice potty training from a young age in a group setting. In many ways the set routine followed in these environments is ideally suited to early toilet training. Although it requires a lot of communication and cooperation, there is no reason to view daycare, or any type of childcare arrangement, as an obstacle to toilet training any more than you would avoid introducing solid food to the baby because the sitter doesn't have a high chair. We find solutions for all of the problems that confront us when we first have children, and you should feel confident that you will find a way to incorporate toilet training just as you have all of those other impossible obstacles that you never imagined your baby would bring.

Timing

Toilet training should closely parallel the introduction of solid foods. By nine months of age most babies cooperate relatively reliably with mealtime. Most parents have developed a feeding schedule that takes into account the baby's personality and desires, and also such practical issues as when it is possible to sit her down in a high chair. Often this is influenced by the caregiver's routines, as well as the needs of siblings and others. Just as you develop a feeding routine that you can (at least usually) stick to at this age, you develop a potty routine that you can fit in to your day.

The best times to start training for most families are first thing in the morning and bath time. When you get the baby from his crib in the morning, try to take him first thing (without much delay, as he is ready to empty his bladder when he awakens) to the bathroom to take that nighttime diaper off, put him on the potty, and sit together for a short visit before you start the day. Often he will void on the potty, or he may have a full diaper and you just get to have a quiet little moment together. From there you can get into the habit of getting him dressed right in the bathroom, or you can follow the routine that usually develops in my house at this age, in which he finishes on the potty and then makes a mad dash to run around naked. This can of course be great fun, and once you have caught him and dressed him you are all ready for your day after an exuberant little bit of time together. All of this play is normal and makes potty time a happy occasion. By building these pleasant associations you are teaching him what a natural and enjoyable thing the potty is. Even if you rarely see results in the potty, that time will come, and you are investing in his acceptance of the process much more than in results at this point.

Alternatively, or additionally, depending on your situation, if you bathe your children in the evening, then make a habit of sitting your baby on the potty right before the bath. This incorporates easily into a bedtime ritual, and the fact that it is usually after dinner makes it likely you will have some success. But your main objective is just to introduce the potty and to try to sit for a few minutes while you talk to her or show her a book or a toy. If she screams, arches her back, or acts distressed, then try again another day. Once again being natural and playful is important. You don't need dancing, singing, bells, or whistles, but you want her to enjoy getting her pants off and sitting on the potty. So be sure to smile and laugh your way through the occasional game of chase-the-naked-baby; let her play and experiment with the whole process.

My boys quickly caught on to the process of using the potty right before bath, and they usually got their business done pretty quickly because they wanted to get into the tub. My daughter, however, had this whole funny game she would play whenever we undressed her for her evening bath, beginning at around thirteen months of age. First she would sit on the potty, immediately get up and look into the potty (which was empty), then go get a book from the shelf, then sit down again, immediately get up, look in, and go get something else, and on and on until she was finally satisfied. She would be furious if you tried to interrupt or cut her short in any way. Initially her little drill did not fit with my plan of getting her ready for bed first, but I learned to get the boys bathed while she did her little thing around us (they found it amazingly hilarious), and then I bathed her last. I can't remember how many evenings I spent watching the boys in the tub laughing hysterically and encouraging their chubby, naked toddler sister to sit on the potty; she would give them a smiling sideways glance and then make a mad dash down the hall, only to return in a fit of laughter and do it all again. Those were great moments that provide the makings of the best kinds of family bonds. I strongly believe that repeated loving and playful encouragement from her family as a part of our regular household routine provided a better foundation for toilet training than any reward system I could have dreamed up.

Sometimes you might get the feeling that spending all of that time in the potty with your toddler is unfair to your other kids who need your attention. My best advice is to involve them. They will learn so much patience, take so much pride in "their" baby's accomplishments, and be exposed to a whole new world of family caretaking and intimacy that you will find it all worthwhile. My kids are close in age to one another, but the encouragement, patience, and love they have shown to one another when someone else's potty needs (or accidents, at times) interrupted what they were doing has been unbelievable. I think kids develop character from daily experiences, and teaching your kids to be patient with a smaller sibling, especially when they can have the wonderful experience of seeing the baby succeed as a result of their help, is one of the best character builders out there.

Most of all, remember to be flexible. It is the hardest part for those of us managing busy lives and busy households, but there really is more than one way to do things. Just think to yourself, when your kids are being playful with the potty, of how many parents have told you stories about their three-year-old refusing to sit on the toilet. They missed out on letting their inquisitive baby discover what fun it could be.

Bowel Movements

Bowel movements are another excellent opportunity for introducing the potty at this age. Many children are quite regular at this time, and you know that they usually stool right after breakfast or lunch. Try to take advantage of that regularity to sit the baby on the potty at that time. The position of sitting is ideally suited for passing stools, and if he takes a moment to relax you will be amazed at the results. Both you and your baby will be much happier to flush a bowel movement down the toilet than to use up a dozen wipes cleaning his bottom after a stool in a diaper.

If he becomes flushed or starts grunting, take him to the potty and sit down with him. I will even interrupt a meal at this stage if I see the baby straining in the high chair, because it is such a great opportunity to familiarize him with the potty. No question, it is incredibly inconvenient to get up from the table and go sit in the bathroom with your baby while your dinner gets cold, but I have found that these are golden opportunities, very likely for success and leading into a lot of interest in using the potty. A baby quickly discovers that it is more comfortable to pass a bowel movement sitting on the potty than lying (or standing) in his diapers, and it is not uncommon for a child begun in this way to crawl over to the potty for bowel movements. There might be occasions when you see him straining, take him to the potty, and then end up with a dirty diaper, a mess in the toilet, and what feels like a mess all over the place, but even this situation goes a long way toward building an association between the need to have a bowel movement and going to the potty for the baby, and it should be handled in a calm and positive way. You will save a lot of money on wipes, and your baby's bottom will be so much better off for it.

If your baby tends to have relatively hard stools or spends a lot of time straining, you should take her to the potty after meals to facilitate easier and more regular bowel movements. It is very important to pay attention to hard stools and to change your baby's diet or discuss other alternatives with her doctor if her stools are frequently hard. Constipation is not only uncomfortable, but it may also lead to future problems, and it certainly interferes with successful toilet training. I discuss this in detail in

Chapter 8, but keep it in mind throughout your training process.

What About Rewards?

There is no reason to offer a reward to your child for sitting on the potty at this stage. In fact it is counterproductive because your goal is to make sitting on the potty a normal part of his routine. When he does void or stool on the potty, it is appropriate to be pleased, but it should be an equal success *whenever* your baby seems to cooperate and is happy to sit and relax for a moment or two on the potty.

What Can You Expect?

The early initiation of potty training follows one of a few patterns. Your baby may act very uncomfortable and irritated, and you should not be discouraged. Keep at it from time to time, but be patient for her to be comfortable with the process. Remember that before disposable diapers were available, mothers had a much stronger motivation to encourage sitting on the potty, and most did so with lots of patience and love. Your goal at this stage is to fall into a pattern where your baby reliably cooperates with sitting on the potty. If she seems comfortable and content, then you start to build on that framework and move into Phase 2.

Possible Scenarios

SCENARIO #1: You introduce the potty at six months of age. You sit your baby on the potty and show her a little toy or a book several times a day. She seems happy and content, and this seems like all of your other interactions with her. She begins to have regular bowel movements on the potty (brought on by the position, or your knowledge of her schedule, or your observance of her grunting or straining and taking her to the potty). She starts to occasionally have some urine in the potty, and one day you can see on your baby's face that she realized that she went, and she will want to get up and look into the potty (and be pleased with herself). You are ready to get out of diapers and get serious about practicing.

SCENARIO #2: Your baby does not sit well until after seven months of age. Even then, he does not like to be unstable and is unhappy to sit on the potty. You should continue to sit him on it very briefly, either in the morning when you are changing his overnight diaper or in the evening as part of preparation for bath. Make sure he feels the security of your arms and knows that you won't let him fall. If he cries, then bring him right into your arms, soothe him, say "That's okay, baby, that's the potty," and go on with your activities. Don't try to make multiple attempts every day until he starts to seem comfortable sitting there and can stay put for a minute. If you see him grunting, then you should take him right to the potty, as he is most likely to be willing to sit there for a bowel movement. When you see that he is stable and comfortable, you are ready to start practicing.

SCENARIO #3: You have an active baby who is already crawling well at six months of age. He loves to be on the go and hates to sit still. If you sit him on the potty, then he lunges forward and literally tries to crawl away.

You should observe him and determine the time of day when he is most cooperative and less distracted. Find something that he thinks is interesting, and save it only for the potty. Keep trying on those opportunities that seem best to sit him on the potty, and if he lunges forward, hold him and hug him, say "Let's sit on the potty," and sit him down one more time. If he lunges into your arms once more, try again later. An active kid can be really discouraging to train because you feel that there is no way he is ever going to sit still long enough to go potty. But it is really important to keep the potty a familiar part of your routine for that very reason. He has to learn to be patient with it, and the more that he is used to taking (very short) breaks from what he wants to do, the more likely you are to eventually have success.

SCENARIO #4: Your baby is happy to sit on the potty and cooperates with multiple trials a day. The problem is that she never actually uses the potty. Often you take off her diaper after naptime, you are so excited that her diaper is dry that you bring her right to the potty, she will sit there for five minutes and be delighted with the three board books you show her, and then the minute you give up and get her dressed she wets her pants. Don't worry. This is totally normal and you should not gauge your success by how often these early attempts are successful or whether she seems to "get it." The objective here is to make her comfortable with the potty so that she can succeed when she is ready. These kids usually do great with early training, as one day it all falls into place. Keep doing what you are doing, and do not be frustrated. Your introduction to the potty is going well.

Phase 2: Practice

(Nine Months to Two Years of Age)

After the first birthday there should be at least one time a day when your baby expects to sit on the potty and knows how to do so. Many love to sit there (and get their caregiver's undivided attention) so much that they want to do it all of the time. Once the potty is an established part of the baby's routine, it is time to start practicing more. This is the part that takes a real commitment from all of the caregivers. You need to provide as much structure to your baby's schedule as possible, and that includes having him in his familiar environment(s) as much as possible. This can be a big challenge to busy families.

Taking Time Out

Often I find that talking to the parents of a toddler about toilet training leaves them feeling overwhelmed and even criticized, in the same way as telling them that macaroni and cheese and fast food should not be the staples of their child's diet. The demands placed on parents in our culture to keep up with the neighbors, to have their kids in all the right activities, and to somehow be in two or three places at once have combined to create an ever-present sense of personal inadequacy. Things like diet, exercise, bowel habits, and overall health are the foundations of living long and well and should be among our first priorities when raising children. If that means that we have to change our lifestyles to allow more time for these fundamentals, then we should seriously look at our options.

Our lives are so busy that many of us feel relieved if we make it through another day with everyone in our family somehow getting fed. Another pediatrician mentioned to me that he saw some results of a survey on eating habits in teenagers that showed the majority of them did not eat any food (over the course of a given week) that required using utensils. Think about that. That is a lot of pizza, burgers, burritos, packaged snacks, and not much else. If they are anything like the teenagers that I see in the office every day, they rarely ever sit down to eat, much less with a family member or friend, and they consume most of their food in the car or in a rush. Not only does this make for bad food choices and obesity, but it eliminates one of the oldest and best parts of human relationships—eating together. Of course the same pediatrician telling me about the study has a home where he and his wife work full-time, and they have an overweight teenager who refuses to eat anything but Taco Bell. He is looking for answers just like everyone else and struggles with what is really important every day. The formation of eating habits starts very early in childhood, and there is no question that that is your first and best opportunity to make a difference for your child.

You should think about potty training in the same way. If your child is having trouble with bowel or bladder control or simply can't catch on to on-the-go potty training, you should not hesitate to alter your lifestyle to support her through the learning process. Keeping up with frequent trips to the potty, while dealing with a toddler who gives you very short notice and often has accidents, can be a huge burden when away from home, and the stress that this creates for already overstressed parents can be significant.

There is no reason to feel criticized, guilty, or like the standard to become the perfect parents is becoming increasingly impossible to attain. We just need to realign our priorities, and understanding why potty training is important is the first step toward figuring out how to make time for it. Remember that this is a very short period of time. Experienced parents frequently attest that their children's preschool years flew by like a moment. Invest all you can in making a solid foundation of good habits in terms of health and diet.

In my family, potty training acts almost like a circuit breaker. There is that constant pull to new commitments, we get stretched too thin, and then someone reaches the age for toilet training. We all make the decision to slow down and start to spend more off time at home. Everyone has to decide what is really important in terms of activities (including Mom and Dad). It is a great opportunity to eliminate some of those activities that you are running to (and working so hard to afford) that nobody is actually enjoying. It is *not* a great time to start a home improvement project or to sign up to head the PTO at your first-grader's school. There are many years ahead to get involved in those things, and a toddler at home is a perfectly good reason to say "I'm sorry, but I can't get involved this year." At the end of the day if you are feeling less overwhelmed and stressed, then you will be more able to calmly deal with an accident and offer just the right kind of encouragement. Your toddler will thrive with a little more predictability and familiarity in his life and his potty training will take off.

Ways to Practice

At this stage, it is a wonderful habit to have your child start to sit on his potty next to you when you use the bathroom if you are comfortable doing that. As an added benefit it is a great way to keep track of an active toddler while Mommy or Daddy goes potty. It does create a lot of work to constantly take his diaper off, let him sit down, and then get him dressed again many times a day. But this is an important part of the process and should not be avoided. You should never say to a baby at this age who asks to go potty "You just went," even if that is true. You must listen to him (and teach him that you are going to listen to him every time) to allow him to learn to listen to his own body. The whole process requires patience, repetition, and encouragement.

As you encourage him to sit on the potty more frequently, you will rely on his overall schedule to determine the exact pattern of when and how often to sit. It is great to start to have a story on the potty before naps and then again when he wakes up. You can begin to have a bathroom ritual before meals that involves going potty and washing hands before eating. If you are changing a diaper, take a moment to sit your baby on the potty before getting dressed again. The idea is to set a routine that you can stick to most of the time. It should definitely incorporate sitting on the potty at his daycare or sitter's house, ideally with the same sort of routine. Gradually build up the number of attempts, depending on how things are going. At first it will be two or three times a day, and by the end of this stage it may be every two to three hours. The trick is to recognize the times in your schedule when it is natural for you and for your baby. Instead of cleaning up immediately after meals in the kitchen, go to the bathroom, sit on the potty, wash hands and face, and change any clothes that are dirty. Look for those types of associations and opportunities.

Getting out of Diapers

Depending on the child as well as your preferences, around one year of age is a great time to start spending some time out of diapers. Spending a few hours in cloth training pants or with a naked bottom contributes a lot to the toilet training process. Inconvenient as it may be, nature intended babies to get the signal that they are wet or soiled, and this process is definitely prevented by disposable diapers. The more that children get the signals from their bodies and recognize the patterns and intervals that go along with their routines, the more their potty training will succeed. Parents who have used cloth diapers know that a baby in cloth will demand to be changed as soon as he is wet, and that pattern of wetting and getting cleaned certainly plays a role in the small infant's developing awareness of the process. Putting him in ultra-absorbent materials such as modern disposable diapers that pull the moisture away from his skin immediately without a diaper change or any human interaction is a different experience altogether.

Some experts have argued that disposable diapers interfere with potty training starting at birth, and that is true to some extent. Signals to the baby's brain when he is wet or uncomfortable play a role in the development of the baby's awareness of the voiding process, and disposable diapers disrupt this process to some degree. However, keeping a baby in cloth diapers in the first year of life is a truly enormous burden of extra work and inconvenience. My personal experience has been to use disposable diapers in the first year of life because it is more convenient, the baby stays more comfortable, and rashes are relatively rare. I can live with that compromise, but it is ultimately a personal decision, and there are many wonderful reasons to use cloth diapers.

Just as the bottle and pacifier (which are used appropriately in babies) will ruin the teeth of a two-year-old, disposable diapers work great for keeping infants' sensitive skin away from their frequent dirty diapers but make it more difficult for older children to succeed at toilet training. The resulting delays can be damaging to the child's urinary system and overall development. The key to successful disposable diaper use, like the use of pacifiers and bottles, is to know when to stop using them and to move on. This should definitely happen within the second year of life. I usually start putting kids in cloth underpants around the first birthday, using a waterproof cover at first. There are many waterproof products out there, but the idea is to get some nonabsorbent cotton underwear or training pants against your child's skin, and then put on a waterproof cover if you want to avoid frequent leaks. It is important to be careful about this, because you want to change her pants right away when she wets. If she is wearing a waterproof cover, you might not know as quickly. So it is certainly preferable, when possible, to have her just in the cotton underwear, so you know immediately when she wets and you can get her to the potty and make that immediate association as much as possible. But a waterproof cover is a great tool when accidents are frequent, as long as your child does not stay wet in them for long. I love Dappis because they are much softer than other plastic pants, but there are several great products out there. We will still have disposable diapers around for nighttime, long trips, or other specific situations. But my goal is to have the baby start to feel those wet pants and learn the signals and timing involved in going potty. The more often that you can have him in cloth pants, the better. Yes, you will have some extra laundry. But you will save some money on diapers, and it is so much better for your baby. It also makes you (and your child) much more likely to sit on the potty if it involves only pulling down pants and underwear, not messing with a diaper and then wondering if you should put that same diaper back on or get a new one. To eliminate any odor, soiled underwear should be emptied into the toilet and then rinsed in a diluted vinegar solution if you are not going to wash it right away.

It is hard to generalize an exact moment when you should eliminate diapers, but birthdays provide a useful guidepost. When your baby turns one he is probably established on a diet of solids, starting to walk, and even using some early language skills. It is wonderfully supportive of his development and all of his achievements to get rid of the bottle, remove pacifiers, and begin to eliminate diapers at this time. It is fine to use a gradual process, but don't stretch it out so long that it becomes confusing to your child what he is supposed to do. Many children at this age will start to take their diapers off themselves, begin refusing bottles, and start wanting to feed themselves. We should recognize and honor this emerging desire for independence and offer our children every chance to succeed. Some parents find that their one-year-old still seems a lot like a baby, really loves his bottle and pacifier, and is reluctant to eat anything other than a few pureed foods. This is not a big deal, and you should not feel that it represents something concerning your child's personality or adjustment. You should be flexible and responsive to your baby, and sometimes that means putting off a big change for a few weeks until he seems more open to it. Use your best judgment, talk to your doctor, but make sure that *you* are not the one who wants your child to keep doing baby things, or that you are not holding on to these habits out of convenience (such as "It's so easy to put him down to sleep with a bottle," "It's so easy to quiet him at the store with a pacifier," and, most central to this book, "Disposable diapers are so much easier").

Daily Routines

It is important to incorporate potty time into your daily routine at this stage, even if it seems that your child does not "get it" at first. A typical pattern for a baby at one year of age is to wake up in the morning, go to the potty, and get changed. If you spend some time playing or doing work around the house in the morning or if she is at a regular sitter, then the morning is a great time to spend awhile in cotton training pants. If accidents are frequent, then a waterproof cover for her training pants is fine. There are a lot of waterproof training pants available in new materials that aren't as bulky and uncomfortable as traditional rubber pants. You should remember that the more time that she spends in cotton pants (as opposed to diapers or Pull-Ups), the faster she will be trained, and the fewer accidents she will have (over time). So try to keep her in underwear as much as possible.

If she tends to have a bowel movement after breakfast, make a trip back to the potty after breakfast. Otherwise aim for a few trips to the potty over the course of the day, depending on the routine of care. Do not *ask* the child if she wants to go. You simply do as you do many other things and say to her "It is time to go potty." You would not ask your two-year-old "Do you want to get dressed for school today?" because you know the answer will probably be no. Instead you have a set routine and you and she know when it is time to get dressed.

When you do have her in diapers, or if she has an accident in her training pants, then try to take her into the bathroom to get changed and have a short sit on the potty while you are there. Of course you know that she already went, but occasionally she will try to hold her urine when she feels that she is having an accident, and then she will finish off on the potty, and you will continue to reinforce the association. I put a towel on the floor in the bathroom and clean her up if that is necessary, and then dress her and send her on her way. The more that you take care of all of her toileting needs in the bathroom, the better it is for the whole process. Besides, have you ever seen an eighteen-month-old who likes the changing table?

What Can You Expect?

This stage has multiple goals. The first is to teach your baby that part of his routine needs to be to go potty.

Learning how to expect and handle these interruptions in his activities is an essential part of his development. The second is that it feels much better to go on the potty than in his pants. This comes quite quickly and naturally to most children at this age if they are exposed to the options. The third goal of this stage is for your child to establish an increasing awareness of his body's patterns, and to encourage him to be conscious of the need to go potty before it happens. He will start to be curious about what comes out of his body, and it is important to develop a vocabulary in your house for all of these wonderful events.

The practicing phase is when your baby becomes a little more predictable with toilet training routines and can often go for long stretches without accidents. But accidents are definitely part of this stage, and knowing how to handle them is an important part of the process. When you first notice that your baby has wet or soiled his diaper or underwear you say "It's time to go potty" and (if possible) take him right to the potty to get cleaned up. You should encourage him to sit down on the potty, even if he obviously just emptied his bladder, because this helps reinforce the association between going potty and the potty itself. I strongly advise against saying such things as "Oh, no, you are all dirty" or "Why didn't you go to the potty?" because he is still learning, and these types of comments make him nervous, upset, and even mad, none of which are very good for the process. Just get some clean pants on and get back to what you were doing before it happened, and make adjustments in your potty routine if necessary.

Possible Scenarios

SCENARIO #1: Your eighteen-month-old baby is cared for in the home. She goes potty when she wakes up in the morning and after breakfast. She wears cotton training pants, and you put a waterproof cover on if you are going out. She sits on the potty about every two to three hours and whenever you think she might need to go. She sits on the potty right before going to bed, and you have eliminated the habit of drinking a large amount of liquids right before bed. She is starting to tell you when she needs to go potty, and she wants dry clothes right away if she has an accident. Your goal now is to start giving her a little independence. It is perfectly okay to continue to remind her to use the potty frequently, but start to give her the skills and confidence to do it herself. Make sure she is in clothes that she can manipulate, and even if you are right there with her let her get her pants off and back on by herself.

SCENARIO #2: Your twenty-month-old baby goes to a sitter or a daycare center. You put her on the potty when she wakes and then again after breakfast if she eats at home. She goes to daycare wearing cotton training pants and a waterproof cover. The sitter puts her on the potty every two to three hours, as well as when she awakens, after meals, and before naps. Every attempt is made to get her changed as quickly as possible when she wets. Your goal is to make everything as routine as possible, but you also need to focus on teaching her how to communicate her desire to use the potty. The more that she can let them know, the more assistance she will get when away from you. You should make sure that you use the words a lot, such as "Let's go potty," "You did a good job going potty," and "We'll try to go potty again soon." She is starting to go potty independently at home and is having increasing success with going potty at daycare.

SCENARIO #3: Your eighteen-month-old baby is at the sitter or else frequently away from home running errands with you. It is very hard to get to the potty as frequently as recommended, and you are frustrated and discouraged. She complains right away when she wets her training pants, but most of the time you are not in a good position to respond and get her changed right away. This is probably the toughest situation, and it is the one faced most commonly by at-home moms who have more than one child. You modify the plan however you can to fit your commitments. If you can devote some time to training in the morning when everyone else is at school, then be intensive during this time and make frequent trips to the potty. If you are around the house after school, then try to use that time to juggle potty training with dinner preparation and homework. At the least get her out of diapers and into cotton training pants, and start to change her every two to three hours, even if you can't make it to the potty that frequently. This provides the basic framework for her to learn to use the potty. You can usually incorporate sitting on the potty as part of your bathing routine without changing around too many things, and you can take her with you when you go to the bathroom.

Sometimes older siblings can get involved, and believe it or not this can be great family time. My four-year-old son would sit with my one-year-old daughter on the potty and read her a book, she would be thrilled and transfixed with his attention, and I got to tell him what an amazing brother and friend he was to his sister. Don't underestimate your older kids and their desire to be caregivers within the family, and you will be surprised at how much they thrive with a little responsibility and trust. My kids are too young for me to claim success at sibling relationships, but when I see my son's tenderness and patience with his sister during these daily tasks, and I see her gratitude and admiration for him, I believe they are building a lifelong bond.

Phase 3: Good Habits
(Between Twelve Months and Three Years of Age)

Most children trained with this plan will start to become reliably dry before their second birthday. Accidents are a normal part of the process, but you should notice them dramatically decreasing by this time and recognize a pattern for going to the potty that works for your family. It is definitely time to be out of diapers. If accidents are frequent, put some waterproof pants over his underwear. It is completely counterproductive to have a two-year-old child in disposable diapers of any kind. If you find yourself thinking it is easier and more convenient to leave him in diapers than to struggle with often fruitless trips to the potty at inconvenient times, then you should think how your two- or three-year-old must feel. He may want to be potty trained, but there are always so many other important, interesting, and fun things to do. You have to show him that you have the patience and the endurance for the task for him to know that he has them, too. If he learns that he can easily return to his play after a potty break, then he will be much less resistant to going.

Many children can go potty on a schedule long before they can talk, and they never have accidents. Others have to grow and develop much more before that happens. As is discussed in later chapters of this book, there are many children who continue to have accidents for many years, regardless of method of training used. It may start to be obvious to you between eighteen and twenty-four months of age that your child seems to have a lot of accidents no matter what you do. You should discuss this with his doctor.

It is well established that prolonged wetting accidents are much more common with boys than girls. The topic of accidents is discussed in detail later in this book. The best way to deal with this problem is to stay with the program, to stick to an established schedule of trips to the potty to try every two or three hours, depending on your child, and to constantly remember to encourage your child not to worry or be distressed, that his time will come if he keeps trying. Even children who are right on target with their potty training achievements will occasionally have bad days, or even bad weeks during which they seem to be falling into a pattern of frequent accidents. You should take it in stride, with a little extra consideration about your child's schedule and routine.

People sometimes say that children are not trained until they go to the bathroom independently without being prompted or reminded. This is a ridiculous idea, comparable to the suggestion that a four-year-old should eat all of his meals without any parental oversight. Childhood is a long process, and part of good parenting involves continual consideration of good eating and sleeping habits, and it also may include an occasional reminder to use the toilet when it is an appropriate time, for many years. For that matter, if reminding someone to use the toilet at a convenient time really suggests that that person is not fully toilet trained, then I know a lot of husbands who are in big trouble with their wives for doing just that every time they get in the car.

Overall you expect a trend toward more independent trips to the potty after two years of age. It is preferable to dress your child in clothes that he can manipulate himself, but he will still usually require some assistance. Remember to teach him to clean himself and wash his hands. If you let him have some naked bottom time occasionally, then he will have the thrilling experience of doing it "all by himself," and this will encourage him and feed his natural desire for increasing independence. You hold on to those good habits of routine trips to the potty upon awakening and before bed (after all, isn't that what you do?), and you make sure everyone gets a trip to the potty before heading out the door.

It is necessary to develop a system for using washrooms in public, no small endeavor for a mom or dad concerned with cleanliness and an active and uninhibited toddler. But you do some very good hand-washing, and for the good of your child you get through it. I advise my patients to keep an extra potty in the trunk of the car to help with some of these situations (as well as road trips), and that can be a helpful alternative when away from home.

The benefits of early toilet training are described and discussed in detail in this book and include many medical as well as practical advantages. It is a labor-intensive process, and it requires a lot of communication among caregivers. It *will* take longer to potty train your baby starting before a year of age than it would to train him at three years old. That fact should not discourage you.

Many people in pediatrics have told me that disposable diapers are just too convenient and no one has the time to spend on more labor-intensive training. This is the same kind of thing that was said when the movement within the profession to start strongly advocating breast-feeding was gaining momentum. People asked that if the majority of women return to the workplace after having a baby, then is it really fair or helpful to encourage them to breast-feed when it is next to impossible for them? The reality is that once the benefits of breast-feeding became well known, many women found a way—they lugged their breast pumps around with them, sat in closets or restrooms to pump off their milk for their babies, stored their milk at the office, transported it back home, and got their caregivers to give it to their babies. Now this is an incredibly widespread practice that is even gaining support in corporate America as some large corporations have created private areas for lactating women. So I think we should be cautious about making judgments about what people are willing to do for their children if they understand the benefits. Furthermore, it is paternalistic in the worst sense to suggest that we won't advocate this method of training because it is too inconvenient for all the working parents out there.

The rewards for this investment include not only the pride and satisfaction in your two-year-old as he masters this task but also several well-established health benefits such as the proper function of the urinary system, less frequent urinary tract infections, and increased bowel regularity. Additionally, you will avoid leaving your baby in diapers that interfere with both his development and socialization. Your potty training memories will include a sweet and often funny set of experiences with your baby instead of a stressful power struggle with your toddler over a new set of expectations. You will find that with love, patience, and a little extra work your baby will thrive in ways you never imagined.

What Can You Expect?

This stage is all about maintaining the good habits your child has already learned. You should continue to focus on her dietary habits, and pay attention to any problems she may be having with constipation. As you are definitely less involved in the process by this time, you may have to do some careful questioning and observation to keep on top of both bowel regularity and overall bathroom hygiene. An occasional daytime accident (wetting, that is) is common and should not cause a lot of concern, even up to five or six years of age. The scenario is usually that your child is really involved in a new activity or is in a strange place, and accidents just happen. If your child starts to have a lot of accidents after being reliably dry for a long period of time, then you need to go see your doctor to make sure that there is not something else going on.

You will see increasing desire for independence, and most children will at least experiment with asking you to "leave them alone" in the bathroom by three years of age. Some children prefer privacy in the bathroom and will even insist on it. Remind them about their hand-washing (setting a good example is your best tool here), and practice their wiping with them occasionally to make sure that their hygiene is good. It is all right to remind kids to go to the bathroom from time to time, but by now their good habits should serve them well.

There are as many scenarios of successful completion as there are children. If your child takes over his own toileting needs before three years of age, never has accidents, never gets constipated, and gets annoyed if you try to remind him to go potty, then leave him be. Allowing children to have the right measure of independence that suits their disposition is an important part of parenting. If your child needs to be reminded to go potty before bed, then that is perfectly okay to continue to do. Some children may want and need your involvement well into the school years, with reminders to go potty before a soccer game, before getting in the car, even when you walk by a public restroom in a convenient place. They will (eventually) develop the maturity to plan ahead and recognize these opportunities, but it is perfectly normal to continue to help them along the way. You know your child, and you should be flexible in defining success as the point when you have a system that works for you and your child, allows him the right measure of privacy and independence, and ensures that his hygiene and bowel habits are the best that they can be.

starting
later

The parents of a three-year-old boy come into the office for advice about toilet training. They read several parenting books over the past two years and have been waiting for readiness signs to emerge. He doesn't seem to have any interest in the potty. He has been growing normally, has a large vocabulary, and can run and kick a ball. He plays well with other children and is generally an active but cooperative child. The parents got him a potty recently, but he refuses to sit on it. If they insist, then he throws a tantrum and demands a diaper. He goes behind the sofa to have a bowel movement, and when he is through he asks to be changed. His parents have offered him everything from stickers to candy to toys to try the potty, but he still refuses. The parents are frustrated, and the preschool he just got accepted to will not take him in dia-

pers. *They are afraid that they "messed up," even though they followed all of the advice out there. They want to know if it is too late to do things right.*

Whenever parents ask me if they missed their chance, my answer is an unqualified no. Parenting requires so much flexibility and responsiveness that there is always the opportunity to change your approach. If you have been holding out for readiness signs, but your child has not shown interest in the potty, then the most important first step is to relax and let go of all of your assumptions and any (misplaced) fears about your child's intelligence, personality, and communication skills. Remember, she does not need to pass any tests before she can sit on the potty. It is not an ominous or even a concerning sign if she shows no interest, is impatient, or even outright refuses. She is engaged in a power struggle with you (a normal part of development at this age), and you must play the part of the adult.

The first step is to make your expectations as clear to her as possible. Avoid saying things like "I don't want to change your diapers anymore" or "You are not a baby anymore." Instead, focus on what a great accomplishment it will be when she can do this all by herself, what a big girl she is, and that you are so proud of her and all of the amazing things she can do. Remind her of all her family members and friends who wear underwear and use the potty. Children at this age have a tremendous desire to imitate their peers, as well as adults, so you want to emphasize that she will be joining this group and be able to do all kinds of interesting things when she is using the potty.

You will go through all three stages of the plan—from introducing the potty, to practice, to good habits (pages 81–115)—just as you would if you started at a younger age, with one big difference: Instead of a baby who is learning to master a new task, you have a toddler whose main focus is being in control of what is going on around her. You should get rid of the diapers from the beginning and start putting her in underwear. Avoid a big struggle or conflict over this important step. Be very matter-of-fact, and show her that the diapers are all gone and it is time to stop getting them at the store. With some children it helps to let them "throw away" the diapers, as this gives them a sense of control and finality. If accidents are frequent, then get some waterproof pants to put on over her underwear and a waterproof mattress pad for nighttime. There are many amazing products out there that are nothing like old-fashioned rubber pants but can go on over cotton underwear and protect your chairs, carpet, and sofa from accidents.

It will help your toddler avoid so much frustration to put him in clothing that is easy to remove. Elastic waistbands on pants are the only way to go, and you won't believe how much more cooperative your child will be with training if he doesn't need your help to get his pants off and on. You don't have to be perfect, but try to think about it when you are shopping for clothes and dressing him, especially when you send him to daycare or preschool, where there are fewer people to attend to his needs. Having an accident while standing in the bathroom because you couldn't get your pants down is just about the most frustrating thing that can happen to a preschooler, and it can cause a lot of resistance and anger with the process. More and more I am seeing larger sizes of children's clothing available with snaps between the legs for diaper changes. Don't buy things like that for your two- or three-year-old. He is naturally developing a desire to do things himself, and making that impossible for him is totally wrong. It even helps if he can easily get his own shoes off (if they slip on or close with Velcro), because many children like to take their pants all the way off to go potty.

There was a rule at the preschool I sent my first son to that the children could not wear anything (including shoes) that they could not get off and on themselves. I had to change just about everything he owned, but I saw how much he loved doing things himself, and how he hated when I tried to lay him down and dress him as I did when he was a baby. It changed the way I buy everything that my kids wear in this age window.

Of course there may be some tantrums, but you can avoid getting into a battle. Make sure she knows this is not any kind of punishment but really a wonderful, exciting thing and that you love her very much. If you are firm and patient, then she will soon give up on the idea of getting any more diapers and you will be able to move on. Of course it might be a rough day or two with a frustrated kid and parents, but it passes quickly and diapers are an impediment to training older children in so many ways. Just as you may feel that you are taking away the greatest comfort from your baby when you stop giving her the bottle, you may feel that you are adding pressure and stress to your toddler when you stop buying diapers. But know that you are projecting your own feelings onto your child with these ideas. I have seen so many parents in the office look at me with disbelief when I suggest one of these changes. I have heard everything from he won't eat, sleep, or get in the car without his bottle. Some parents insist their child is unable to sleep except in her parents' bed. When I am in doctor mode all of those things sound ridiculous, and I try to explain that babies at this age are really adaptable, and they won't resist a change that you have made in a clear and consistent manner for more than a day or two.

As a parent, I know a day or two of conflict with your child over bedtime, bottles, pacifiers, or diapers seems like an interminable, intolerable, and unnecessary misery. I can only say that I have seen it play out hundreds and hundreds of times, and the children are so much better off when their parents are making active (and sometimes tough) decisions about these things. You need to be in charge, to know what is best for your child and why, and to follow through with it with patience, love, and above all consistency. Of course you don't want your child to stop needing you, to grow up too fast, or to feel that you pushed her or abandoned her in any way. But if you watch and nurture her natural curiosity and desire for independence ("Do it *myself*, Mommy!"), then you will see that these baby things, when used well beyond their necessity, obstruct normal development. With time you will see that the independence from these things leads to mastery of the tasks that serve as the foundation of confidence for things to come.

Many parents have told me that they feel it is unfair that many preschools demand that children be potty trained before they enter school, but naturally I completely disagree. I have seen children who are in diapers at three years old in a preschool environment with other toddlers, and it is amazing how much less confident they are with everything from socialization to actual learning. The other children treat them like (and often call them) babies, and the whole situation does not work out. Of course there are exceptions, and some children cannot be reliably trained at this age. You must individualize not only your own expectations but also the type of environment that you place your child in for care. The last thing that you want to do is start him in preschool with a stigma that makes him instantly aware that the other children are doing something that he feels he can't do. To succeed he needs to feel secure, and to feel secure he needs confidence.

As you start to put him in underwear, begin to build a routine that fits with what you already do. Wake up in the morning, and go to the bathroom with your child. He should sit on the potty, wash his hands, and then have breakfast. If he resists, say "Okay, we'll try again later." There is no need to insist, argue, scream, threaten, or force him to sit down. If he wants to run around with no pants on, I think that is fine, but it is really up to you. You can certainly feel all right about insisting that he has pants on in your home if that is your choice. If he cries for a diaper, then show him that you don't have any more, that it is time to wear underwear. If there is a tantrum, then treat it as you would any other tantrum. Try to talk to him and comfort him, and if there is no progress, then walk away for a few minutes and tell him you want to talk to him when he is finished crying. Repeat this as many times as necessary, but keep your patient, calm, and reassuring manner.

As I have already explained, there are many factors that

determine how frequently your child needs to use the washroom. It is probably less than ten times a day, but it depends on habits as well as bodies. Once she is in underwear you will start to get an idea of how frequently she goes, and you can develop your plan from there. To stay dry it may mean a trip to the potty every two hours, or three, or it may be enough to use your cues such as meal, nap, and transition times to go potty. The big difference when introducing the potty to an older child is that she has developed a desire for control and independence, and it is natural for things to develop into a power struggle. To avoid this try to refrain from discussing and negotiating. You do not ask a two-year-old "Would you like to have breakfast, or do you just want to go outside and play?" Likewise, you should never ask if she would like to go potty. Just as you say "It's time for lunch," you must say "It's time to go potty" and avoid any question about whether she needs to go. This is where it is particularly helpful to couple the potty with other things such as "Let's go potty and wash our hands before dinner," or "Let's go potty before we get your shoes on to go." And she will see it as part of the routine steps necessary for transitioning from one activity to another.

If he is really in the middle of something, but you know that he needs to take a break or else run the risk of an accident, then reassure him that no one will disturb his work or play. If there are other children around, then offer to put his toy or puzzle where no one else will bother it while he is going potty, put a marker or name tag on top of it that the other children will not disturb, or tell him "Daddy will watch your toys for you while Mommy takes you potty." It is so important for him to learn that he can feel secure leaving something that he is enjoying to go potty and that everything will be right there waiting for him when he is finished.

Finally, remember that the older she is, the more stressful accidents become. Friends and siblings may start to make fun of her when she wets or soils, and she will be very sensitive to this. You must casually reassure her. Accidents are not a big deal. All children have them sometimes. It is not horrible or stressful or disgusting, and you should let your child know that is how you feel (even if you sometimes don't). Be prepared, so that you can get her clean and dry and quickly back to play. The less that she fears accidents, the less stressful the whole enterprise becomes. It is totally normal for things to be going great, to have no accidents at all for a month, and then to have one every day for a week. If your child is otherwise well, and things are normal at home, just take it in stride, keep that extra set of clothes on hand, and make sure she is getting to the potty frequently.

In most cases toilet training older children goes very quickly once they are over their resistance. So your main focus is to be loving and kind, but you must also be firm that there simply are not going to be any more diapers. Set a routine that you can all live with, and require your child to sit on the potty on that schedule (regardless of results). Remind him that he is just practicing and that it is okay if he doesn't have to go. Be patient, and avoid a power struggle by being as matter-of-fact as possible. Remember, resisting toilet training is a lot like a tantrum, and the more attention that you pay to it, the more that the child learns that it is a good way to get attention. Short-circuit the process by giving him your positive attention and praise and not focusing on problems with toilet training.

toilet training children with special

F
I
V
E

needs

SCENARIO #1: *The parents of a two-year-old bring him in for a routine visit. He is growing well, but his parents are concerned that his development seems to be behind other children his age. He will imitate a "mama" sound but does not use any words independently. He will occasionally point to something he wants but otherwise does not communicate. He will not follow a command to get a ball or a toy and does not seem to understand the household routine. He only recently began to walk and still seems "clumsy." He is easily frustrated and throws a tantrum when he is dressed or put in the car. He is not interested in toys and does not show much curiosity about household objects. His play is very repetitive, and he resists the introduction of new activities. He does not seem interested in other children and seems to ignore them in social situations. The parents want to know what to* expect from his development, and how to know if he is ready to be toilet trained.

SCENARIO #2: *The parents of a three-year-old boy who has been diagnosed with developmental delay come to me for a regular checkup. The child is enrolled in speech, physical, and occupational therapy. He had a hearing test that was normal. He saw a pediatric neurologist who did a set of blood tests to check for genetic and metabolic problems and an MRI and EEG of the brain. All of these were normal, and there is no history of developmental delay, autism, or mental retardation in either family. He has shown some improvement with his therapies and is now feeding himself with a spoon and helping to dress himself. He does not use any words or appear to respond to any questions or direction, but he does know a couple of signs that he uses frequently. He is in diapers, but his parents have sat him on the potty a couple of times without success. Everyone has told them to forget about toilet training for now, but they are wondering if there is any possibility that he could be trained.*

Toilet training often seems like the least important thing to parents who are going through all of the grief and adjustment involved in the (often gradual) realization that their child is not developing normally. It is particularly hard in the preschool years, because it is difficult to predict what a child with developmental delay without a known cause will be like in the future. Many people are working very diligently on this topic to be able to distinguish significant developmental delay in the first few years of life from the normal variants, or late bloomers, who eventually catch up and are completely normal.

Often, especially with early intervention and intensive therapy, children with significant developmental delay in the first few years of life can do amazingly well in the school years. All pediatricians, developmentalists, psychologists, and therapists remember the preschool-age children that they assessed as having the type of developmental delay associated with severe mental retardation or autism, only to have that child make amazing strides and prove them wrong. With our current level of understanding about developmental delay in the preschool years, the best advice many parents are given is to arrange for a full evaluation of their child (including seeing a developmentalist, neurologist, and a geneticist, if possible), get as much therapy for him as early as possible, and wait and see.

Given all of this uncertainty, and the fact that you are usually working without a clear diagnosis or even clear expectations about your child, how do you make decisions about toilet training? Clearly it is a very individualized process. Once developmental delays have been recognized it is important to make sure there is not a diagnosis such as a chromosomal disorder, metabolic disease, or abnormal brain development or brain injury that could possibly have some specialized treatment or at least offer you a better sense of what you can expect in the future. Motor development, including a full evaluation of any muscle weakness or stiffness, should be included in the evaluation. This can be done best by a pediatric neurologist, but there are many physical and occupational therapists that are excellent at recognizing these types of problems in very small children. In many cases no cause for the developmental delay is found, and the parents must confront the fact that their child's future is uncertain.

I had a great teacher in my residency whose patients had some devastating disabilities. When parents pressed her for some kind of picture of what the future might hold, she would try to gently skirt the question. If they insisted on an answer, then she had this response that always knocked the wind out of me when I was in the room: She would say that the only thing that is certain for any of us is death, and that she gave up trying to predict that long ago. She would say very plainly that you just make a plan, and know you are going to change it as you go along and put one foot in front of the other. And we would all just sort of stand there in the exam room, thinking, Lovely, how helpful, that didn't answer their question at all. And I remember being annoyed that she wouldn't go out on a limb at least a little and tell them what she thought was likely.

But in the end, after I became a parent and felt the real vulnerability and loss of control that comes with loving someone that much, I started to understand her message a little better. I have adopted my own softer version of it when faced with difficult questions from parents about what to expect in the future with their child who is not following a normal developmental trajectory: We don't know what the future holds for any of our children with any certainty. You have to exist with a highly individualized combination of hopeful optimism, denial, and preparation for the most practical problems that you might face to make it through parenthood at all. It is unfair that some parents are confronted with this painful fact at a time when most parents are still getting really upset about their child getting a bad haircut. You need to get through those evaluations, start all of the therapy, and see what happens.

Because our toilet training guidelines have centered for so long on the language skills of the child, many parents of developmentally delayed children have been advised that the whole project did not concern them because their child does not talk or in some cases does not communicate at all. This has been such a point of frustration for me as I read all of the literature about this topic. There is absolutely no reason to think that language or communication skills are necessary to embark on a toilet training plan. Experts have proven this with institutionalized adults with severe mental retardation or dementia. Using a regimented toileting plan, many of these adults have become reliably clean and dry. Numerous plans utilize sign language, some use pictures on cards as cues and prompts, and some use dolls or other models.

Drs. Nathan Azrin and Richard Foxx created a plan for developing continence in institutionalized patients back in the 1970s that centers on using the toilet on a schedule. Their plan has helped hundreds of people, whom many said could never be dry, become continent. A psychiatrist I know told me a story of an adult patient of his who was institutionalized with severe dementia who suddenly got very agitated and needed to be restrained while he was in the middle of treating her. They were considering medicating her until she urinated on the table and then calmed. When her aide returned for her she said matter-of-factly that it had been time for her (the patient) to use the washroom.

How many people out there are still in diapers because no one has taken the time to recognize (and make a plan for responding to) their signals? I firmly believe that no matter what the degree of mental incapacity, no one should sit in his own excrement if it can be avoided. We should definitely not assume we can determine if a certain person "knows the difference."

So that brings us back to toilet training your child with developmental delay. Once you have had the tests and seen the specialists deemed appropriate for a full evaluation, and you have your plan for intervention in place, it is time to think about toilet training. The age is less important than when you think your child might be able to cooperate. In some children you know that there is no possibility they will sit down on the toilet, and in those cases you have to wait and continue with the other therapies. But if you see any possibility of implementing a routine of sitting on the potty at certain times or at certain intervals, then you should start doing it just as you would for any other child. Get her into some cotton training pants and introduce her to the potty. Try to develop a routine that can be incorporated into her therapies, if appropriate.

You can model toileting behavior yourself, with videos (there are many animated videos that demonstrate children using the potty) or by using dolls. This can be particularly useful in children without verbal skills but who can learn complicated things through observation. You may want to teach your child a sign for potty, or give her a note card with a picture of a child (ideally herself) sitting on the potty that she has access to. I have seen some therapists who work with children with autism use this technique in kids without verbal skills to teach them to communicate their basic needs. Basically you make an area where you have a set of note cards with photographs of the child doing things like eating or drinking or sitting on the potty. When she is frustrated or agitated, you direct her to the board and try to get her to look at the cards to see if she can identify what she wants. With time your goal is that she will go and get the card that pictures her on the potty and then show it to you as a means of communicating her needs and desires.

In the end it is going to be completely individualized, and you will have to trust your instincts. Virtually all of the therapists out there now have been trained to keep children with developmental problems in diapers unless they meet the readiness criteria. So if you approach your child's speech therapist, he will probably say that your child can't be toilet trained until his language skills improve. Your child's occupational therapist may say that he can't be trained until he has better fine motor skills and coordination. You might not get a lot of support for implementing a toilet training plan.

Many group-care centers and schools are more aggressive about training and will be willing to work out a schedule with you, but you may have to be a real advocate for your child. If you find that your child is able to sit on the potty at home, then you should really push for her other caregivers to start to incorporate toilet training into their school and therapy schedule. You will have to work together to make a plan that can be consistent and, hopefully with time, recognizable to your child. Try to take every possible opportunity for your child to wear underwear (a waterproof cover is fine). Even children who have no communication abilities can better sense wetness if they are not in disposable diapers, and they may start to hold their urine to make it to a set potty interval.

Sensory integration problems, which are present in all children with mental retardation as well as in all autistic children, can work both for and against you with toilet training. On the one hand the child's unique sensitivity to tactile sensations can make some of these children eager to be dry and no longer require you to wipe their soiled bottoms. The converse is that these problems make anticipating the need and recognizing the urge to use the washroom especially difficult. My advice is to give your child a trial out of diapers with scheduled trips to the toilet. If he seems distressed or uncomfortable, then try a more gradual approach, like just trying to sit on the toilet after meals or before bath.

As with normally developing children, constipation and stool withholding will disrupt any attempts at toilet training. Do not hesitate to make a big deal out of your child's constipation with your doctor, especially if effecting dietary changes is out of the question. Some children with autism or mental retardation are particularly sensitive to different textures and strong flavors and can tolerate only a very specific diet. There are medications available that can help keep these children regular, and you should not let your child remain constipated, even if everyone is telling you that it is the least of your concerns.

In the end you will be able to see what works for your child. Remember to have an open mind to the fact that working on conditioned behaviors (such as simply sitting on the toilet on a set schedule for a child who cannot communicate) can really lead to total continence. And consider all of the communication tools out there and give them a try before you determine that your child would never understand the doll that voids or a picture of a toilet, for example. Children with special needs surprise us all of the time with discovered abilities that were never observed or recognized until some thoughtful person tried something new.

some common problems

UNDERSTANDING,
PREVENTING, AND
DEALING WITH TOILET
TRAINING PROBLEMS

P
A
R
T

3

bed-wetting and accidents

The parents of a healthy four-year-old girl bring her in for a regular checkup. Her growth is normal, and she has been doing well in preschool for the last year. She can write her name, recognizes many letters, has an extensive vocabulary, and plays well with other children. She began toilet training at around two years of age and seemed to "do fine" except for the occasional accident and frequent bed-wetting. She has had many dry days but has never been reliably dry. Her parents are concerned because she wets her pants almost every day at school. They put her in a Pull-Up at night, and they aren't sure how often it is wet. She uses the bathroom independently most of the time with few reminders, has never had a urinary tract infection, and seems moderately upset by accidents. The parents are considering putting her in Pull-Ups for school to make accidents less noticeable. They have tried many reward systems to keep her from having accidents and have punished her on a few occasions when she seemed to have an accident on purpose, or right after they asked her to use the bathroom. They want my advice about what to do next.

Many people express a concern that early toilet training leads to more frequent accidents and bed-wetting, and I want to discuss this topic in detail. Once again definitions play a central role. If you consider an accident any time the child wets underwear but not a diaper, then of course earlier elimination of diapers will seem like more accidents. In converse if you leave your child in diapers longer, then he will wet his underwear less. But that does not mean, as it is often said, that putting him in underwear and beginning toilet training *caused* him to have accidents. If you define accidents as any time the child goes somewhere other than on the potty, then he will have accidents much more frequently and for prolonged periods of time the longer that he is kept in diapers, as described by the increasing ages of training.

Every parent dreads being caught in public when her child yells out "I had an accident!" especially when you realize that you don't have a change of clothes for her. My three-year-old once looked at me in such a situation, with all of the other parents we were with looking on, and declared "Mommy, you are supposed to have clean pants for me in your bag." I have tried every possible solution to get out of this situation, from stripping him down and discreetly pushing a half-naked child in the stroller to the car, to removing soaked underwear and putting his shorts (just a "little wet") back on, to (and this is true) taking the shorts off my younger child and leaving him in underwear so I could put his shorts on his older brother. I don't advise doing these types of things, as I can tell you your kids will be pretty mad, and you will feel lousy. Actually, the number of times I have faced a public accident with my kids has been quite few, but obviously I remember those occasions, my frustration, embarrassment (a little planning on my part could have avoided the whole thing), and sympathy for my distraught child.

Many parents delay toilet training to avoid these situations, and it is important to put accidents in perspective, before you let your fear of them determine your potty training plan. If you teach your kids to be calm, be prepared, and take accidents in stride, then they will be much more comfortable with the whole process. I remember that sinking feeling when I picked my son up at preschool and saw him in different pants than I had dropped him off in. I knew that he must have had an accident, and I was sure that he was going to be really upset about it. Of course the first thing he said to me was "Mom, I had an accident today and everything was in my cubby, except I didn't have clean socks, so could you get me some?" I felt triumphant (except for the forgetting the socks part) because he was so calm, unaffected, and practical about the whole matter. I had a confident, resourceful kid who was not going to let a little accident ruin his day. In many ways I view that moment as one when I felt most successful at potty training, even though I had a bag of wet clothes to wash.

Bed-wetting and day-wetting accidents (jointly referred to in medicine as enuresis) are problems that have existed in childhood throughout recorded history with remarkable consistency. It is more likely that genetic traits contribute to this occurrence than the changing trends in toilet training. It appears in most studies from different time periods and cultures (all reflecting different training attitudes and techniques) that a similar proportion of children struggle with bed-wetting at different ages. There are thought to be several contributing factors to one child's risk, some of which are well understood and treatable.

The History of Wetting

In the 1950s Dr. Lucille Glicklich compiled a thorough review of the historical literature on enuresis going back to antiquity. Her paper is fascinating and often hilarious as it describes the many remedies for this problem throughout the centuries, and a few are highlighted below. The important message from all of this is that this problem has always existed—in every society regardless of toilet training methods, parenting styles, environmental and cultural influences, or degree of stigma attached to it. Although it is sad to think of the many children who have undergone painful or humiliating therapies throughout history for a problem they would have soon outgrown, it is more unconscionable that we fail in our modern society with our expansive knowledge of these systems and sophisticated diagnostic tests to properly understand, diagnose, and treat these children.

Enuresis has caused concern since the time of the Egyptian text the Papyrus Ebers, dated 1550 B.C. It contains a remedy for the incontinence of urine that consists of juniper berries, Cyprus, and beer. Throughout the Middle Ages, various saints were believed to offer cures for this problem. The medieval scientist Paulus Bagellardus published the first printed book on diseases in children in 1472. The twentieth chapter of his book was called "On Incontinence of Urine and Bed-wetting." He states:

> Parents are especially saddened as a result of bed-wetting when either boys or infants beyond the age of three years continually pass water in bed, and this sometimes not only within the space of a single day or two days, but continually, every night, and not only to the age of five or six years, but sometimes beyond the time of puberty. This is said to be very base and in a certain measure unfortunate for the boys thus born.

Bagellardus goes on to describe many commonly prescribed remedies including administration of the cerebrum of a hare, the flesh of a ground hedgehog, and the comb of a cock, as well as the application of a plaster made of lung of a kid. In 1544 Thomas Phaer published his *Boke of Chyldren*, which is recognized as the first book on pediatrics written in English. In the section entitled "Of Pyssing in the Bedde" he describes a remedy made by mixing the trachea of a cock, the testicles of a hedgehog, and the claws of a goat.

Increasing knowledge about human anatomy and physiology is reflected in the eighteenth-century writings of Thomas Dickson. He advocated the application of blisters to the sacrum (tailbone): "As most of the nerves which go to the bladder pass through the foramina of the os sacrum, I thought it probable that this might be of use." He describes the case of a thirteen-year-old girl with enuresis who was treated with the application of a large blister to her sacrum. Dickson reports the girl was cured within twenty-four hours.

Medical writings in the nineteenth century reflect an explosion in scientific discovery and understanding. It was clearly established that there was a familial tendency toward enuresis. The musculature of the bladder was described as two systems, one being the detrusor, which contracts or empties the bladder, and the other being the vesical sphincter (which is actually part of the detrusor), which contracts to close off the bladder, thus preventing it from emptying. From early in embryonic development the bladder contracts and empties at regular intervals. At no point with a normal baby does urine simply continuously leak out, and this process of voiding at relatively predictable intervals is part of our inborn physiology.

Multiple theories emerged linking enuresis with either an overactive detrusor or a weak sphincter. The neurological system was thought to influence enuresis by several distinct mechanisms. As a result of malfunction of the nerves going to the muscles of the bladder, those muscles might contract or relax in an uncontrolled manner. Additionally, the nerves from the spinal cord might fail to convey the information regarding the state of the bladder to the brain.

An important development occurred with the writings of Dr. George Phillippe Trousseau in 1870, in which he argued that enuresis was the first in a chain of neuroses. He believed that a person might suffer from enuresis as a child and later in life develop hysteria, epilepsy, and finally insanity. The possible connection between epilepsy and enuresis was discussed for many years until ultimately discredited.

Finally, laziness and obstinacy were suggested throughout the years as possible causes of enuresis in children. Samuel Adams refuted this with complete clarity on the subject in 1844:

> None of the brute creation will lie in their urine if they are not tied or penned; then why do we attribute this practice in the rational being to laziness? Simply because some are not able, by a careless and superficial examination, to find the cause, and well knowing that their reputations will be at stake if they do not account for the act, they too often condemn the helpless child to daily floggings.

Adams's statement sounds particularly profound in light of the developments of the twentieth century. Although medical science continued to explore human physiology in all other areas, the psychoanalysts dominated the discussion of enuresis. Even as new advances in understanding about the role of brain chemicals (called neurotransmitters) in such disorders as depression, anxiety, and attention problems led to new medical therapies for these problems, enuresis continued to be attributed to psychological (rather than physiological) causes. Dr. Clifford Sweet argued in the *Journal of the American Medical Association* in 1946 that enuresis is based on one or any combination of three conditions:

A. The child has not as yet matured with reference to bladder control; or those who have acquired it do not know how to use it. They have been poorly trained, under tension or with lack of parental sympathy or understanding. As a result, the child has become bewildered, tense and thus retarded with reference to bladder control.

B. Subconsciously, the child wished to remain in or return to the irresponsible state of infancy rather than assume the normal dangers or responsibilities of his age. This may be aroused by jealously of new siblings, feelings of insecurity and inability to resolve a conflict such as disagreement among parents.

C. Subconscious resentment against parents.

Dr. Leo Kanner's book *Child Psychiatry* was published in 1948 and further advanced the idea that enuresis was connected to psychological disturbance. He states that male enuresis results from identification with the father as urination symbolizes ejaculation and fulfills the subconscious desire for potency. Enuresis in the female child, he argues, is an expression of the unconscious desire for masculinity (once again with urine somehow psychologically representing semen). These ideas are so bizarre, and so out of touch with modern science, that it is alarming to see how much they have contributed to the current guidelines.

Dr. William Sears also addressed the issue of bed-wetting in the 1950s. Put into the context that the children in this study were trained much earlier than is commonly done today, the results are interesting. He reports that 44 percent of the children in the study had no bed-wetting since two years old or earlier, 22 percent had none since three years old, 6 percent stopped at age four, and 10 percent had occasional bed-wetting after five years old. His data clearly showed that the age of beginning training had no influence on the possibility of bed-wetting in a given child. It did show, however, a relationship between the severity of the toilet training process and late bed-wetting.

Different studies reflect varying numbers relating to bed-wetting. Dr. Kirk Weir collected data from 706 London families in 1982. There is no information in his study reflecting training techniques. He did note that the prevalence of wetting was much higher than in comparable studies, of interest as most of the children were presumably trained with disposable diapers and modern techniques. This study tried to link certain factors with the children who had continued wetting. The following factors were associated with day-wetting: sex (boys more commonly wet than girls); bed-wetting (bed-wetters more likely to day-wet); soiling (children with stool accidents more commonly have day-wetting); developmental score (standardized number based on questionnaire negatively associated with day-wetting); language development (weak association between delayed speech and prolonged wetting); and behavior problems (also from a standardized questionnaire, very weakly associated at this age). Factors that were shown *not* to influence wetting included social class, housing conditions, anomalous family composition, family size, birth weight, body size, general health, admissions to the hospital, family life stresses, child's social contacts, relationships with siblings, and nervousness.

You often hear parents swear that their older child had increased accidents when a new baby was brought into their home, there was a death in the family, or there was any other stress in his life. By definition any change may affect toileting habits if it is built into your child's routine. But if children do have accidents as an outlet or externalization of stress, then the phase passes quickly, and it is best not to focus on the symptom. Instead offer him as much stability and reassurance as possible. In fact you probably become much more aware of occasional accidents that would not have even registered in your memory banks otherwise when *you* are feeling stressed and overwhelmed. So try not to attach so much significance to accidents, and avoid asking "Why is this happening?" because it will probably pass in a few days or weeks, and it is best if you keep up appearances of routine around the house. The key is to try to return your child to his schedule (or establish a new one, if you need to) as soon as possible.

The definition of enuresis has changed over the years, as well. Today approximately 82 percent of two-year-old children wet the bed occasionally (not specified), going down to 49 percent at age three, 26 percent at age four, 20 percent at age five, 10 percent between the ages of six and ten, and about 3 percent in the teenage years. These numbers are considered normal, so by definition it is usual for some children to have prolonged bed-wetting. The American Psychiatric Association's *Diagnostic and Statistical Manual* defines enuresis as two or more accidents a month in a child between five and six years old and one accident a month for a child more than six years of age. There is no distinction made in the diagnostic criteria in boys and girls, despite the fact that all studies show that enuresis is much more common among boys. Rates of bed-wetting overall in four-year-old children are found to be 12 to 30 percent in studies from multiple Western countries and 10 to 16 percent in six-year-old children. Of the children still without dryness at night, for each year from the age of five about 15 percent will become dry. Bed-wetting also clearly runs in families, and about 50 percent of children who are bed-wetters had at least one parent who had the same problem. Children whose parents were both bed-wetters have a 70 percent chance of having the same problem.

In 2000 a group of Belgian urologists reported success in treating voiding disorders in older girls that were associated with urge symptoms, enuresis, and frequent urinary tract infections (UTIs). Their program was based on creating a voiding and drinking schedule and learning the proper posture (with foot support) for voiding. They remarked that their methods were very similar to the more regimented toilet training techniques that were popular in their country forty to fifty years before. They suggested that the more frequent problems with lower urinary tract in children (including frequent urge to void and recurrent UTIs) might be caused by improper (or inadequate) modern toilet training techniques. The authors argue that more structured (scheduled) toilet training might be beneficial as a way of avoiding later bladder instability.

The Importance of Anatomy

If your child has ongoing wetting problems, then you should have her evaluated by a physician to ensure that no other (often treatable) problem exists. I have seen several children in the office who were thought to have accidents because of a behavioral problem, only to be discovered years later to have an abnormal urinary system. For example, a ureter can implant into an abnormal location during embryonic development. A little girl I saw in residency had this problem (called an ectopic ureter), and it caused urine to leak (uncontrolled) from her vagina. For years she was thought to have frequent accidents, and her pediatrician even sent her to a psychologist at one point because he felt it was a behavioral problem. Finally, when she was seven years old, she developed a serious urinary tract infection that led to imaging studies being done of her urinary system. Once the problem was found she underwent surgery and returned to a normal life.

Although these types of problems are rare, it is very important that you know that everything is normal with your child medically if he continues to have frequent accidents despite good efforts and cooperation with training. This is especially true if he has had *any* urinary tract infections (whether someone called it a bladder infection, kidney infection, or urine infection does not matter). Once it is established that your child has normal anatomy, physiology, and development, behavior management can be implemented to treat enuresis. This is an area in which earlier, more regimented potty training is far superior to the readiness approach. When urologists treat children for enuresis, they utilize a structured method that relies heavily on biofeedback. To put it simply they put the children on a schedule that involves drinking extra fluids, making frequent trips to the toilet, and ensuring they are in the right position to optimally control their muscles.

The human body is designed so that our best defense against infection of the urinary system is frequent emptying of the bladder. When we urinate we effectively wash out any bacteria that may have made it to our (normally sterile) bladders. The longer that we hold urine there, the greater the possibility of these bacteria gaining a foothold and causing an actual infection that can lead to damage or scarring of the urinary system and occasionally to serious illness. We should keep this fact in mind when we are teaching our children potty habits. It is a good idea to drink plenty of fluids for many reasons, and having a healthy urinary system is a big one. Part of toilet training young children is encouraging them to drink fluids, make frequent trips to the washroom, and avoid waiting for an urgent need to go before emptying their bladders.

The "residual volume" is the amount of urine left in the bladder after we urinate. You can visualize it as the amount of fluid remaining after you pour out a glass of water into the sink and then set it back down. It is normally a very small amount, but there are several disorders of the urinary system that lead to a high residual volume (meaning a lot of urine is still left in the bladder after the person feels finished urinating). These conditions predispose to more frequent urinary tract infections, for all of the reasons discussed. This is important for parents to understand because residual volumes are much lower in children after they are toilet trained. In effect the bladder is more successfully emptied when the child tries to go on the potty than when she goes more randomly in a diaper.

A group of Swedish doctors found that children with a bladder disorder associated with poor emptying experienced a marked improvement in their residual volume after toilet training. Put another way, children whose bladders were not emptying properly when they were in diapers were found to empty much more normally once they were toilet trained. Given all of the problems and concerns associated with urinary tract infections, the fact that the more that children hold urine in their bladder the more likely they are to have an infection and this tendency can be resolved with earlier toilet training leads to a significant argument for such training of all children.

There are several chemicals made by the body that regulate the amount of urine the body produces. The function of the whole system is to remove certain waste products from the body and to maintain a proper balance of fluids and electrolytes. The human brain monitors both our blood pressure and the level of electrolytes in our blood. It sends a chemical called antidiuretic hormone (ADH, also known as DDAVP) to "tell" the kidneys to produce less urine (or to conserve water for the body). The kidneys also have a built-in system to regulate the amount of urine produced based on salt concentrations, and the body has several other hormones that regulate urine production, but this (amazing) system is beyond the scope of this book. DDAVP is particularly important to understand because a medical formulation of it is commonly used to treat bedwetting. If children who continue to struggle with frequent bed-wetting after five years of age respond to a medication that is a substance naturally made by the body, then isn't it possible that the reason that they have the problem is that they have a naturally low level of this substance? So if giving a child DDAVP stops his enuresis, then the reason that he had it in the first place may have been a relatively low level of DDAVP. The fact is that it is really not known what causes most children to have wetting, but there are numerous points in our physiology that may be proven to play a role and provide treatment options in the future.

Another variable that affects enuresis is sleep patterns, as arousability varies among individuals. If your brain is simply less responsive to stimuli when you are sleeping, then you will miss the signal to wake and use the toilet more frequently. Finally, behavioral patterns vary widely with respect to the issue of fluid intake and voiding patterns at night. Many people learn from a young age that they cannot tolerate drinking fluids in the evening without waking to void. For some this idea is never instilled or practiced.

The Importance of Learning and Habits

Children must be taught to use the toilet when it is convenient and not to wait for the most critical moment, when finding one may not be possible quickly enough. It does not come naturally to them to do things that we as adults routinely do to avoid discomfort and inconvenience. You do not find yourself extremely thirsty right before bed, then drink a huge glass of liquid, then use the washroom several times overnight. Instead you naturally drink plenty of liquids throughout the day, regulate the amount of fluids you drink right before going to bed, and limit sleep disturbances. Throughout the day you use the bathroom before getting in the car, leaving for a meeting, or going to the store. You are not applying pressure when you teach your children to do the same. This idea is central to the plan of toilet training that is presented in this book. Allowing children to determine when they use the washroom, without teaching them that they should get in the habit of going at convenient times throughout the day and that there is some planning involved, is setting them up for failure, frustration, and possibly toilet training resistance and prolonged accidents.

Treatments for Enuresis

The most effective treatment available for prolonged bedwetting in children is the use of a nighttime alarm that awakens them with a beep or a vibration when they wet. Numerous products are available that utilize this principle, and doctors have used them for many years to treat children with problematic bed-wetting. Most consist of some sort of pad that you put on the child's bed that sets off an alarm if she wets while sleeping. The alarm causes her to wake up, realize that she wet, and get cleaned up. The process is one of conditioning, and with time most children using these devices begin to awaken before they wet. They work very well, and most parents find you don't have to use them more than a few weeks or months before children stop bed-wetting completely. Doesn't the fact that these alarms work so well make the practice of using Pull-Ups on all preschoolers at night seem like a bad idea? If training the body to not wet while sleeping involves some signals (like waking up because you feel wet) that teach the sequence of when wet, wake up, get dry, go back to sleep, then aren't we undermining the process by removing those signals?

Often parents report that they are still putting their four-year-old in Pull-Ups because their child wets the bed at least once a week. In many cases they are open to using an alarm to wake the child when he wets or trying antienuresis medications. It makes so much more sense to give the child a period of time during which he goes to bed in regular underwear and then you can keep track of how often he voids. Frequently the stress and frustration associated with (usually everyone) getting up when a child wets the bed will lead all involved (including the child) to be more aware of how much they drink before bed, and will also train them to arouse before voiding. While alarms are a great tool, they should not be used before the child spends at least a few months limiting fluids before bed and is sleeping in regular underwear. Nature provides the alarm when the child feels cold, wet, and uncomfortable. You should give him a chance to learn from those signals (in a supportive and absolutely nonpunishing way) before trying an external alarm.

Significantly, as cited in the *British Journal of Urology* in 2002, a group of doctors also looked at the prevalence of behavior problems in children both with and without enuresis and found no differences between these groups. The authors also looked at family background and found that there was no difference between the group of children with wetting problems and those without in terms of coming from a first-marriage family, a one-parent family, or other situation. So we need to question all of our assumptions that prolonged wetting represents some sort of acting out against problems at home or disruptions early in development.

The Special Case for Girls

A special situation sometimes occurs with little girls who seem to be doing well with potty training but frequently have wet underwear. The parents often tell me that it seems that their daughter wets a small amount in her pants shortly after she goes on the potty. If you notice this happening, then you should see your doctor because there can be more than one explanation for this problem. In most cases, however, the problem is reflux of a small amount of urine into the vagina. This can easily occur when girls rush to finish at the potty. That small amount of urine that flowed into her vagina while she was urinating will leak out as she runs and plays and will often look like an accident. If this happens frequently, then you should make a point of slowing her down a bit in the bathroom. You can tell her to sit still and count to ten after she is finished going potty and before she gets up, or to look at a book, or to do any other habit that will make her sit still for a few extra seconds to ensure that her bladder is empty and all of the urine is out of that area.

Girls need a little extra attention in general when potty training, as proper habits and hygiene from a young age can prevent many uncomfortable episodes of vaginitis. They must wipe from front to back to avoid spreading all of the germs from the rectal area around the vagina and urethra. It is also completely normal for girls to have their hands in these areas at times, and caregivers should focus on teaching proper modesty, appropriate public behavior, and (above all) good handwashing. Many girls can't tolerate sitting in the bathtub for long periods of time without getting a lot of irritation in the vaginal area, and if it becomes an ongoing problem, then switching to showers is a great alternative. I usually tell parents to use whatever bath products they want, but the first episode of skin, bladder, or vaginal irritation means it is time to be more careful, and the initial step is to stop all of the bubble bath and other bath products, to use a mild soap to cleanse her body, and to get her out of the tub as quickly as possible.

All of the evidence shows that the urinary system should be trained from a young age to function synergistically to empty the bladder completely at regular intervals. We should not teach children to rely on urgent signals from their bodies that they are getting uncomfortable before they go to the bathroom. As an adult consider how often you wait to get really uncomfortable before you empty your bladder. It happens on long trips or in certain situations, but in the course of a normal day you go to the bathroom long before you feel a sense of terrible urgency. It is an important and almost totally overlooked part of toilet training to teach children to do the same. The secondary benefit is fewer accidents when you don't rely on your child's sense of timing and planning to make a trip to the potty.

urinary
tract
infections

It is important for all parents to understand urinary tract infections. They are frequently misdiagnosed and mismanaged by healthcare providers, and the consequences can be serious and lifelong. There used to be a distinction made between a bladder infection (called cystitis) and a serious kidney infection (called pyelonephritis). As it stands now this distinction appears to be unimportant, if it even exists. The urinary system is supposed to be sterile (free from bacteria) from the bladder all the way back up to the ureters and the kidneys. If there are bacteria anywhere in this system, then there is the potential for the infection to spread, leading in the short term to serious illness and in the long term to kidney damage. The standard terminology now is to refer to all infections of this system simply as urinary tract infections. The presence of fever suggests that there is more serious illness going on currently, and many medical decisions are made based on whether it is a "febrile" or an "afebrile" infection, but even infections without fever can have long-term consequences.

This is a tricky situation, because in babies and toddlers the only symptom of a urinary tract infection may be a fever, and in some cases there are no symptoms at all. So in pediatrics we are supposed to have a high index of suspicion for urinary tract infection in small children and to consider checking for one any time a baby has a fever or seems ill, especially if there is no obvious focus (like a cold or an ear infection). Whenever a child complains of abdominal pain or painful urination, her urine should be checked. If there is ever a sudden increase in the number of accidents that a previously potty trained child is having, then her urine should be checked. In the first year of life there is a relatively high risk of a urinary tract infection spreading and leading to a body-wide infection (called sepsis) or even meningitis. As a result many babies with urinary tract infections, and probably all of them with febrile urinary tract infections, may need to be hospitalized for close monitoring and treated with antibiotics.

It is essential that your doctor does a proper urine culture before any treatment is begun. This means that when the urine sample is obtained, it should be collected in as sterile a fashion as possible. The external parts of our bodies are covered with bacteria, and if some of them get into the sample, then the results can be very difficult to interpret. So you must clean your child very well and try to catch some urine midstream in the sterile cup. It is always preferable from a medical standpoint to have a catheterized sample (obtained with a small tube put into the urethra), and it really is a quick procedure. No parent enjoys putting a child through unpleasant medical procedures, but you should understand that there are valuable pieces of information that can be gained, which can really help with decision making down the road.

Once you have this sample your doctor can order a urinalysis. A urinalysis can be done with a dipstick in the office, and it can indicate if there are any white blood cells (fighters of infection), blood (often seen in infections), or several by-products of bacteria. It gives a rough picture of the likelihood of there being an infection. At this stage your doctor has to make an assessment based on how ill your child appears, combined with the rough data provided by these initial studies, and determine how to proceed. The options are to order further tests, start medication, or observe your child's illness.

Regardless of the management decision made at that time, you should make sure that some of your child's urine is sent for a urine culture. To do a urine culture a small amount of urine is placed in a culture medium and observed for several days to see if any bacteria grow. If none grow, then the urine is normal (sterile), the urine culture is called negative, and there is no infection. If bacteria do grow, then it is possible to identify them and to determine based on laboratory tests which antibiotics they are sensitive to. Sometimes a culture is called contaminated if bacteria grow that are not typically associated with urinary infections and are common organisms found on our skin. This means that some bacteria got into the culture from someone's hands or else from your child's body when the urine was being collected. It is a good idea to repeat all urine cultures that come back as contaminated to make sure that the urine is really sterile.

The results of the culture are not only important for treating the current infection, but they can also give valuable information about the child's urinary system. Unusual bacteria in a urinary tract infection should alert your doctor to be much more aggressive about considering why this occurred. In my experience any urine culture that grows something other than E. coli bacteria suggests that that child should have further testing done of her urinary system.

We live in an era in which bacteria are increasing their resistance to antibiotics, so knowing the sensitivity of the bacteria causing the infection can be an essential piece of information. Having a urine culture and doing it properly are the only ways to get this information. Make sure that whenever a urinalysis is done on your child, they send some of the urine for a culture, even if you are in an ER or an urgent-care center. You can call for the results, and they will help your doctor make the right decision about further treatment or evaluation over the next few days. Repeated urinary tract infections can lead to scarring of the kidneys and are one of the leading causes of kidney failure in adults. It is extremely important that you have a physician keeping track of any time your child had a urinary tract infection, the organism that caused it, and its antibiotic sensitivities.

In normal circumstances urinary tract infections should not happen at all in children. They do, and often we cannot find anything wrong with the child's urinary system that would explain why. It is, however, very important to look. There are two tests that are commonly used to evaluate the urinary system in a child who has had a urinary tract infection. One is called a renal ultrasound, and it is an easy, painless scan of the kidneys to look for any indication of scarring, enlargement, or dilation of the collecting system that would warrant further evaluation. It involves the same technology used in obstetrical ultrasounds, an experience most parents are familiar with. The second is called a voiding cystourethrogram (or VCUG), and it is a lot less enjoyable to undergo. Compared with a lot of unpleasant tests in medicine, it really is not a big deal, but it does involve inserting a catheter into the urethra to instill some dye into the system and then taking a series of X-rays to observe the dye (where it goes) and how the bladder empties. This information is incredibly useful and important, and you can detect many problems that can be treated *before* there is damage done to the kidneys.

The leading cause of recurrent urinary tract infections in children is called vesicoureteral reflux (or VUR), which just means that urine is going from the bladder back up the ureters toward the kidneys. In normal people, there is no reflux. When it occurs it significantly increases the risk for urinary tract infections and kidney damage. Some of these problems are being picked up on prenatal ultrasound, so the baby can be managed from birth to avoid any of these complications. Most children are diagnosed with this problem as a result of a urinary tract infection. More important, there are several treatment options (from long-term antibiotic use to surgical repair), and most children outgrow the

The Special Case for Boys:
Circumcision and
Urinary Tract Infections

What about boys? Boys and girls are, as we all know, anatomically different. As discussed in the text, in general, girls are much more likely to acquire a urinary tract infection than are boys, with about 8 percent of girls and 1 percent of boys before the age of seven suffering one or more acute infections. Part of this difference is due to anatomy (as the bacteria simply have a longer distance to travel to cause an infection in boys than in girls), and part of it may have to do with circumcision.

According to a recent meta-analysis (a large study that compares the results of many different studies done over the years on the same topic) of studies comprising more than 400,000 patients, around 1 percent of boys get UTIs overall, but there is a significantly higher incidence in uncircumcised infants. It is important to note that the incidence of UTI in boys is so low that it takes a very small number of individual cases to cause highly signifi-

cant differences in risk across the population when statistical analysis is applied, and this certainly is true when looking at the rates of UTI with and without circumcision. The number of circumcisions needed to be performed to prevent one UTI was found to be 111, and the incidence of complications of circumcision was about 2 percent. The authors concluded that circumcision is therefore only medically necessary in boys who are at particularly high risk for UTI (such as boys with urinary reflux or other abnormalities of the urinary system or nervous system).

More important, however, other researchers have shown that uncircumcised males may be at higher risk for more serious complications from UTIs. Researchers looked at the records of 136,086 baby boys born in U.S. Army hospitals between 1980 and 1985. For the 100,157 circumcised boys, there were 193 complications. These included sixty-two local infections,

continued

eight cases of bacteremia (infection of the blood with bacteria), eighty-three incidences of hemorrhage (thirty-one requiring ligature and three requiring transfusion), twenty-five instances of surgical trauma, and twenty urinary tract infections. (Getting circumcised does not guarantee that the baby will not get a urinary tract infection.) In contrast the complications in the 35,929 uncircumcised infants were all related to urinary tract infections. Of the eighty-eight boys with such infections, thirty-two had concurrent bacteremia, three had meningitis, two had renal failure, and two died.

Thus, the risks of complications of the procedure need to be balanced against the heightened risk of UTI without the procedure. It seems that according to the latest research the risks and benefits of circumcision are closely balanced. There are of course other important issues (such as religious and cultural factors) that legitimately enter into parents' thoughts about this subject. I believe that these things in general outweigh any supposed benefit of circumcision in the prevention of UTIs—if circumcision is of religious significance, or a strongly held cultural value, then it is absolutely all right to do. Otherwise your son is probably better off, all things considered, living in the world with all the parts that he came into it with. The numbers of purely elective or cosmetic circumcisions being done in the newborn period are falling significantly every year in this country, and you should not be afraid of your son being different from his peers.

problem completely with very conservative treatment. With proper management, you can prevent any damage at all to the kidneys. Finding those few children who require more aggressive treatment to avoid kidney failure makes all of those unpleasant VCUGs that turn out to be normal worth the effort.

constipation

The parents of a five-year-old boy named Michael bring him to the office because they are concerned that he is frequently constipated. The mother reports that he seems to avoid having bowel movements but will occasionally soil his underwear with small amounts of stool. He was a breast-fed baby and had normal runny stools as a baby. He first became constipated in the toddler years and would frequently cry during bowel movements. His mother used various remedies including glycerin suppositories, but the problem always came back.

Michael's growth is normal, and he is doing well in kindergarten. He was toilet trained at two-and-a-half years of age without any problem or resistance but seemed to "hold" his stool. He was never punished for accidents. He has frequently passed *small, pebblelike stools and on a few occasions had bleeding after a bowel movement. He has a good appetite, but his mother reports that he is a picky eater. He eats pancakes for breakfast, a sandwich or macaroni and cheese for lunch, and chicken nuggets or a hot dog for dinner. He refuses to eat any fruits or vegetables but drinks four or five juice boxes a day. He has always been a big milk drinker and "doesn't like" water.*

Michael's parents want to know if they can use any laxatives and what else they can try to help him. His parents have noticed that he seems to be having accidents of small amounts of watery stool in his underwear, and he insists that he was not aware that it happened at all.

Michael has a textbook case of encopresis. This condition results from long-standing constipation and stool withholding. It leads to dilation (or enlarging) of the large intestine and rectum. Once these structures are stretched for long enough, they stop sensing that they are full. The child does not even feel that he needs to have a bowel movement anymore, and the only way for the stool to get out is to leak around this huge mass of impacted stool that is sitting there. The treatment is to get rid of all of that stool with an aggressive cleaning-out regimen, usually consisting of a series of enemas, a serious change in diet, a program of oral laxatives or stool softeners, and a bowel retraining program. This usually means that he needs to sit down on the toilet after meals for a set period of time (around ten minutes) and just relax. We used to joke in my office that this is the one appropriate use for a Game Boy.

The child just needs to sit there and be distracted so his body can start to work again, and ten minutes of Game Boy usually does the trick. Of course if you prefer to use books or other distractions, then that is perfectly okay.

The cause-and-effect relationship between toilet training and constipation has been debated for years. Many proponents of psychoanalytic theory have argued that constipation results from excessively pressured toilet training. I have even had adults tell me in the office that they believe that they are constipated because one of their parents spanked them when they had an accident in childhood or forced them to sit on the toilet for long periods of time during toilet training. While I don't recommend spanking children (or punishing them at all, for that matter) for accidents or forcing them to sit on the toilet when they don't want to, there is nothing to indicate that it has any connection to constipation later in life.

Constipation is a common problem, accounting for 3 percent of visits to pediatricians and 25 to 30 percent of visits to pediatric gastroenterologists. A universal definition of constipation does not exist, and many people mean different things when they say that their child is constipated. A common scenario in the office is that the parents have brought in their infant because they believe he is constipated. They have been told by all of the nurses in the hospital, by the lactation consultant, and by all of the parenting books they have read that the baby must have at least three bowel movements a day. This is good advice, and monitoring stool production is one of the only ways available at home to see (especially in breast-fed babies) if the baby is getting enough to eat.

I have a few more resources available in the office (like an infant scale), and I need a few more pieces of information from the parents before I can address their concerns. First, has the baby been feeding well, is there any fever, vomiting, or signs of illness? Second, what do they mean by constipation? Once we establish that the baby has gained adequate weight, the answers to my other questions are critical. If the parents report that the baby is doing fine, eating well, and thriving but that she has not had a bowel movement for four days, then I can reassure them that everything is fine and the situation is normal. There are not a set number of bowel movements a baby needs to have each day, and in fact this number fluctuates in most children during the first year of life. Some babies have one regular bowel movement daily throughout infancy, while others have a small stool after each feeding in the first few months and then the number of bowel movements a day gradually declines. Even breast-fed babies can go seven to ten days without a bowel movement, and if they are continuing to eat well, gain weight, and otherwise thrive, and have been evaluated by a physician for other problems, there is no reason for any intervention. Constipation must involve hard and painful defecation and not simply refer to less frequent bowel movements.

If your baby has not passed a stool and is acting uncomfortable, not eating, having fever, vomiting, or looking listless or ill in any way, then you need to call your doctor right away because this does not represent simple constipation. At the other end of the spectrum, if your baby seems uncomfortable and turns red or grunts during bowel movements but passes normal stools, is eating fine, and seems to be thriving in every way, then he is not constipated and does not need any medication. It is very common for babies to have an episode during which they strain or grunt, fuss, and seem to be having trouble passing a bowel movement. I have been in that situation as a mother, and you feel so helpless with that miserable little baby looking at you all red in the face that you are willing to try anything to help. The best thing to do is to try to feed and comfort him, and be patient for nature to take its course. If you must do more than that, then you can use a sliver of glycerin suppository or some lubricant on a Q-tip. It is best to talk to your doctor, and remember to be gentle and use these methods rarely. An ounce of prune juice, Karo syrup, or a teaspoon of mineral oil by mouth will often help as well.

If he is doing well in every other way but passes infrequent, hard, and painful stools that often look like pebbles, then you must make the important distinction between an episode of constipation and a child who is usually or even frequently constipated. If he has frequent episodes of straining, crying, and grunting, and passes hard stools, then he is actually constipated, and it is very important to deal with this problem.

As with enuresis there are several medical problems that should at least be considered in children with ongoing constipation. These problems are very rare, and given that constipation is a common problem, the vast majority of children with constipation do not even need to be tested for these problems. Make sure that you mention and describe your baby's bowel habits to your doctor, and she should be able to determine if anything about your baby suggests other causes.

These organic causes of constipation include Hirschsprung's disease (a disorder of the development of the nerves in the rectum), hypothyroidism (which would be picked up on with most newborn screening programs), abnormalities of the spinal cord (including tethered cord), and imperforate anus (often with an opening elsewhere, allowing the stool to leak out, appearing like normal stools). The main thing that should cause you to consider some of these diagnoses is if the constipation is present in the first few months of life. If your baby has normal stools until solid foods are introduced, then the possibility that one of these disorders is causing her constipation becomes almost zero.

When children make the transition from being an infant to being a toddler, their own and their parents' perceptions about their bowel habits change. They become able to actively hold their stool, and this is the beginning in some children of a cycle of hard and painful stools, followed by an episode of stool withholding in order to avoid that painful stool, followed by soiling episodes. Parents often report that their toddler is so constipated that he goes into a corner, grunts, strains, and can't pass the bowel movement. In many of these cases the opposite is occurring, and the child is actually grunting and straining to hold a bowel movement *in*, either because he does not want to have it in the diaper or take the time to go to the potty, or because he fears a painful defecation. This is why it is so vitally important to avoid multiple episodes of hard and painful stools. Once the cycle of stool withholding is in place, it takes an active effort to retrain your child that bowel movements are not painful in order to break it.

The Effects of Diet

In most children with chronic constipation, the real culprit is diet. Many of the dietary changes that have occurred since the 1950s in this country (specifically a large proportion of our diet consisting of highly processed food) predispose to constipation. Additionally, our weaning practices have changed a lot over the years. With exclusively breast-fed babies, Mom's milk production (and the baby's consumption) decline as the baby starts eating solids in the first year of life. Babies that are bottle-fed from birth have a (virtually) limitless supply of milk provided to them, and many continue to drink their full caloric requirements long after they are eating a regular diet. Not only does this contribute to the obesity problem in American children, but also milk is very constipating. This may seem paradoxical, as most newborn babies have very frequent and loose stools while on an all-milk diet. But as the system matures and the baby begins to have less frequent bowel movements, regularity depends on a balanced diet of solids with adequate fluid intake and decreasing milk consumption.

Once the baby is eating a (sensible) diet of solids, her milk consumption should really drop off. If you do choose to wean to the bottle (as you will probably need to if you are weaning under six months of age), make sure you are not offering the bottle even more than the baby was accustomed to nursing. The calcium and fat in milk are essential for the proper development of babies' bones and nervous system, and the point here is not to deprive her of these vital nutrients. The focus is on how much milk a child should drink at what age, and there should be a significant decline in this amount by the time a baby reaches a year of age and is eating solids.

Stop Giving the Bottle

All babies that are bottle-fed should eliminate the bottle around a year of age. There are several reasons for this. First, they simply don't need it anymore. They are able to drink from a cup and eat solids, and you should encourage their natural curiosity about food and their (increasing) desire to feed themselves. There is an important developmental transition between the liquid diet of infancy and a diet that centers on solids. It does not matter how many teeth they have, because all babies can chew soft foods with their gums. If your baby struggles with textures and chokes easily, then you have to go slowly, but most of these children do well on pureed foods and yogurt until they pass through their particularity about foods. After you get rid of the bottles, your baby can move on to more interesting things like experimenting with different tastes and textures of foods. Continuing to suck on a nipple does not fit into this developmental stage.

Eliminating the bottle completely is one of parents' greatest fears. The most common question I hear is "How will I get him to sleep?" My usual advice is to physically get rid of the bottles at one year of age, go through a set bedtime routine that is familiar to the baby, and put him down in his bed at the same time every night (as much as you can). The truth is that you should never get into the habit of feeding your baby to sleep in the first place, and I think the most helpful piece of parenting advice out there for new parents is to feed your baby, comfort and snuggle him, but put him in his bed while still awake *from the beginning.* He will sleep so much better and easier for his entire childhood. If it is your habit, however, it is time to break it at a year of age, and you may need to listen to a little bit of crying. Like so many other things, weaning *yourself* off of the bottle can prove more difficult than weaning the baby. Those are precious moments, holding your baby in the rocking chair with that milky smell and his contented hum, and they pass too quickly. But new opportunities for bonding with your baby will emerge (I promise), and starting to limit his milk consumption around a year of age involves eliminating the bottle at this time. If he is not given a bottle, your baby will naturally drink less milk.

The second most common fear about elimination of the bottle that parents express is that their child won't drink enough milk. This is part of the argument to eliminate the bottle sooner rather than later. A one-year-old is much more flexible, has a shorter memory and less built-in obstinacy than a two-year-old, and will likely adapt to drinking milk from a cup within a few days. The older toddler may get into more of a power struggle and flat-out refuse to drink milk if you take her bottle away. Better to avoid this situation. If you find yourself in it, be patient, calm, and deliberate. Toddlers lose interest in a power struggle if they don't sense that you are all that interested. Get rid of all the juice drinks and other options, and offer only milk or water. If she asks for a drink, give her that choice. If she says no or has a tantrum, tell her those are the only choices you have and to let you know when she wants one of those choices. Don't start putting chocolate in the milk or make any other alterations. Just be patient, don't argue, and make sure she understands the options. If two weeks pass without any progress, time to talk to your doctor to check on her calorie, fat, and calcium needs, and how you can provide them.

Usually the bottle is a convenience for parents. I ran into this with my third child, who always seemed ready for lunch just when it was time to pick up her brothers from preschool. She wouldn't eat it half an hour earlier, so she would drink her bottle in the car on the way there and be happy the whole time. When we stopped giving her the bottle I had a much less cooperative baby on the trip to preschool, but it passed quickly, and she learned to eat before we had to go. In retrospect it was never necessary to make it a part of our routine to give her that bottle in the car; she could have learned to have her lunch or a snack before we headed out, before she did and probably with a less difficult adjustment. She has certainly never suffered from extreme hunger in her life. But you lose perspective as a parent sometimes, and you just have to tough it out when it is time to fix a problem.

There are several reasons that the elimination of the bottle will help you with toilet training. The first is that you will begin to limit the amount of liquids your child drinks in the evening, which will (eventually) allow him to be dry at night. Parents often complain that their toddler does not sleep well at night, and I always encourage them to think about their child's fluid intake. All babies experience some degree of arousal when they urinate, and as they get older they often completely wake up and cry for attention. When you think about it, would you sleep well at night if you drank a couple of huge glasses of milk right before bed? Limiting evening fluids is a gradual process, and you should certainly let your toddler have as much to drink as he wants. The problem with the bottle is that he is not drinking to satisfy hunger or thirst at this age; he is drinking from habit. If you break the habit, he will drink the amount of fluids that he needs, which I guarantee you will be less than he takes from the bottle. His nighttime diapers will be less full, if not dry, when he awakens, and he will sleep with less disruption. With time he will stop drinking much of anything at night and wake up dry after an uninterrupted night of sleep.

Solids

Additionally, if you get rid of the bottle, you will effectively limit your baby's milk intake after a year of age. This will eliminate one of the biggest causes of childhood constipation. Once your baby is off the bottle (or weaned) and doing well with a solid diet, she should drink around eight to ten ounces of milk a day. Keep her on oatmeal or some other high-fiber cereal for breakfast, along with some fruit. Lunch should involve some whole-grain bread and fruits and vegetables. It is okay to hide the good stuff from kids—putting fresh fruit, bran, granola, or flaxseed into their yogurt, smoothie, cereal, noodles, or sandwich can be a great trick. You can put cheese on their broccoli and pretend raisins are little bugs to eat. Just make sure you are setting a good example with what you eat, and avoid having a lot of sugary snack foods around.

I have seen babies that are hooked on everything from

oranges, dates, avocado, garbanzo beans (by the fistful), frozen peas, dried apricots, silk tofu, sweet potatoes, and baked apples. I have seen a three-year-old (my own) sit at the table and eat five whole pears from a bowl in about ten minutes and devour an entire cantaloupe at one sitting, only to flatly refuse it one week later. With a little faith and creativity you will find things that are good for your child that he loves, and it is normal for him to change his mind frequently about what he likes.

You should use only whole-grain bread and rolls from the beginning. Try to substitute wild or brown rice for white rice, and let him use carrots or apples to scoop up his beloved peanut butter. My two-year-old was happy to lick the peanut butter off of those apple slices that I cut up for him rather than eat them, and I never said a word to him about it. I would eat the apple off of his plate before he got up from his snack. It lasted only a few weeks before he started eating his whole apple and saying "Mommy, you have to get your own."

If she eats packages of snacks all day long, then she will not eat her meals, much less what you want her to eat. A sandwich on whole-grain bread is preferable to anything prepackaged or in a can, and neither more work nor more expensive. She should sit at the table to eat; you need to make a point of avoiding a lot of eating in the car and stroller. It is just as easy to have a box of raisins and a banana in your bag as it is to have a bunch of crackers, and you will be surprised at how easily your child adapts. In this country we give our kids way too much food, and way too much of the wrong food, and you should avoid doing what it seems like everyone else around you is doing. Children do not need

constant easy access to food. More than
ican children are obese (a number stead
the consequences of this trend are stagger

Dental Health

This leads to another reason to stop giving the
year of age. Sucking on a bottle is terrible for b
The sucking motion distributes that sugary liquid
it is milk or juice) all over his teeth, and he holds
mouth much longer than if he took a drink from a cu
may seem like a remote concern when you are look
your little toddler, but you will take him to the de
around his third birthday, and you will feel awful when
dentist finds a cavity. The first thing she will ask you
when you stopped giving the bottle, and if your answer i
eighteen months, or two or (gasp!) three years old, be prepared for a lecture. I am exaggerating of course, and the pediatric dentists I know are really sensitive people, but that is
pretty much what it feels like when you are the parent in
that situation. Remember that dental hygiene starts in the
first year of life.

Additionally, prolonged use of the bottle predisposes children to increased risk for ear infections. The sucking motion
distributes that sugary liquid all the way into the area of the
eustachian tubes and encourages bacterial growth. Children
who are struggling with recurrent bouts of middle ear infections should get off the bottle and start drinking from an
open cup to limit this. For all children, there is a definite
benefit in terms of limiting the number of ear infections to
eliminating the bottle at an early age.

second question the dentist will ask you when she
ds that cavity will be how much juice your child drinks,
d the only right answer is *none*. That sounds a little ex-
eme, but juice is a big part of the constipation discussion
s well as the bottles and cavities discussion, so I bring it up
here. Children do not need juice. They do need fresh fruits,
and pureed versions of them in smoothie form may be the
only way they will eat them. The apple or grape juice you
buy at the grocery store (or fruit punch or lemonade) has
none of the nutrients that make eating fruit a vital part of
good health. Juice is full of sugar and has a very high con-
centration of calories. It encourages a taste and craving for
sweets, dulls the taste and appetite for healthy foods (like
an actual piece of fruit), and encourages the terrible toddler habit of grazing to avoid the tedious task of actually
sitting down for a meal. If you must give her juice, then it
should never be in a bottle and really never be sucked at all
(that includes those spill-proof sippy cups), and considering you do not want it all over your house and car, that
usually means don't give it at all.

Now you are wondering why I would suggest that juice
is constipating, when fruit is so helpful for this problem.
There are two parts to the answer. The first is the more obvious one, that juice does not contain all of the fruit, that it
has no fiber, and there are many beneficial nutrients and
properties found in an actual piece of fruit that do not end
up in the juice. The second part relates to the huge
amounts of juice many toddlers drink, and the fact that
they do not eat a proper diet because of it. It is so common
to hear parents complain about their picky toddler who

would never eat cereal, or whole-grain bread, or an actual fruit or vegetable. When you look at his diet, he is getting most of the calories he needs in the four or five cups of juice he drinks every day. Not only does the elimination of all of these good foods lead to terrible bowel habits, but also these eating habits tend to stick, and it is close to impossible to get a seven- or eight-year-old to eat something he is not used to.

Finally, the habit of drinking sugary beverages follows many children into adolescence. I can't count the number of times that I have sat in the office with overweight teenagers who ask me what to do to lose weight. The first thing I ask about is what they drink, and virtually all of them drink enough soda, juice, sports drinks, and other sugary concoctions to account for thousands of calories a day. Many teens lose significant numbers of pounds simply by eliminating all of those drinks and substituting the eight glasses of water they should be drinking anyway for proper health. We should never start them on this habit, and it starts by keeping them off juice as babies, and instilling a love of fresh fruit by keeping it available, eliminating unhealthy alternatives, and setting a good example by what we eat.

Chronic Constipation and Encopresis

What if you have done all of these things the best that you can and your child is still constipated? There are multiple medical regimens to break the cycle of constipation, but it helps to understand how this system works so you can comprehend the treatment plan. As the stool passes through our intestines, water is absorbed out of it back into our body. The longer the stool stays put, the more water is absorbed and the harder the stool gets. In many cases children get an anal fissure (or tear) from a hard stool, and this makes the subsequent stool very painful. Naturally they learn to avoid painful bowel movements so they hold them in as long as possible. So it is really a vicious cycle. If you are constipated, then you are likely to get more constipated.

These hard bulky stools cause the rectum (which is the final part of the large intestine where the stool is held before being eliminated) to dilate, or enlarge. The nerves that give us the sensation that we need to have a bowel movement are located in the wall of the rectum and are sensitive to stretching or distension of the rectum by the stool. Over time if the rectum becomes increasingly dilated from holding large amounts of stool for long periods of time, then these nerves stop working and you actually lose the sensation to have a bowel movement as well as the control over having one. This results in a condition called encopresis, where there is an impacted mass of stool filling the rectum, and small amounts of watery stool leak out around it (called overflow incontinence) without any ability to control it. Many of these children never have normal bowel movements but instead have frequent soiling of their underwear.

This can be an incredibly stressful and embarrassing problem for the child and the parents. Many will not even mention it to their doctor. In fact it is a common problem, reported in 1 to 3 percent of school-age children. The cause is unknown, but a history of painful, hard stools early in life is common. It has been stated that 50 percent of these children can be treated with an increase in dietary fiber alone, but there are several medications and other interventions available, as well. It is very important for parents, children, teachers, and doctors to know that this is not a behavioral problem. Children with overflow incontinence of the stool have no sensation of it, no warning that it might happen. It is in no way a gesture of defiance or disturbance.

The treatment of encopresis is basically the same as the treatment for chronic constipation. You should see your

Does Your Child Have Encopresis?

1. Repeated passage of feces into inappropriate places (e.g., clothing or floor), whether involuntary or intentional.

2. At least one such event a month for at least three months.

3. Chronological age is at least four years (or equivalent developmental level).

4. The behavior is not due exclusively to the direct physiological effects of a substance (i.e., laxatives) or a general medical condition, except through a mechanism involving constipation.

—From the Diagnostic Criteria for Encopresis from *DSM-IV*.

doctor, and if she seems unfamiliar with a treatment plan, you should be referred to a pediatric gastroenterologist. The goal is to ensure that the child has regular, soft, painless bowel movements, and to prevent any buildup of stool in the rectum so that it can return to a normal size and the sensory nerves in the wall can start working again. You must begin with a "cleaning out" regimen, which usually consists of a series of enemas and laxatives or stool softeners, followed by a maintenance plan centered on dietary changes combined with stool softeners.

To toilet train children in the first year of life, people throughout history have used the fact that children are most likely to stool after eating. If we are seeing high rates of constipation in our society and frequent problems with stooling disorders in children trained with readiness guidelines, then maybe there is a connection. If we teach our children to sit and relax on the toilet for a few minutes after eating, then they will have more regular bowel movements that will be by definition softer and less likely to be painful. This could avoid the initiation of the whole cycle of delaying and avoiding bowel movements and would set them up for a lifetime of healthy bowel habits.

frequently asked questions

N
I
N
E

Won't it take longer to train my child if I start earlier?

When people ask me this question I first ask them what they mean. If they mean that they will spend all of this extra time on potty training and their child will be trained at the same age he would have been whatever they did, then the answer is definitely no. There is ample evidence that children who start training earlier finish training earlier. If the parents are asking if their time commitment overall to toilet training increases if they begin earlier, then the answer is yes. It places more demands on a caregiver to take her baby to the potty and sit there with him than it would to change his diapers until he could handle toileting on his own.

I often hear parents in the office express concerns that

it will "take too long" if they begin training earlier. People have developed a sense that if their child is not toileting without much reminding or help, then they are wasting their time and should leave him in diapers until he is older. Many parents have proudly told me that their child one day "asked for underwear" and then "trained himself" with almost no accidents at all. No child should have to reach the stage of development where he can recognize underwear at the store and tell you that he would want to wear it instead of diapers before you even introduce him to the potty.

Parents should not measure how successful they were at potty training by how little time and effort they invested in it. If there are benefits to the child who has had delayed toilet training, then they have not been reflected in any of the (many) studies done on this topic. The problems with delayed training are discussed at length in this book, and I think there are more than enough reasons to make an extra time commitment to this task.

What do I say to people who tell me I am being pushy by putting my one-year-old on the potty?

This can be one of the most challenging areas of being a parent. We have all faced those situations where we are bombarded with unwanted advice from all sides. Other mothers are often the worst offenders, and I have been guilty of it myself. It is just so hard to keep your mouth shut when the urge to share your parenting experiences strikes. When you find yourself on the receiving end of any comments, either critical or "helpful," try to be gracious. Remember that most people's intentions are good and that they probably care about you and want the best for you. If possible, the best policy is to smile and ignore. If that doesn't work, then you can come up with a polite statement like "We've talked about this a lot and made our own decision," or "I'm glad that worked for you, but this is our child."

Part of my motivation for writing this book was to provide a more definitive answer to this question, or at least make parents feel more confident with their decision. I have seen so many families with the intention of potty training in a traditional manner be pressured to wait by their friends, or sitter, or neighbors, or family members. If you have someone insisting that you are making a mistake, then my hope is that this book has provided you with the specific and concrete tools to explain the basis for your plan. Most of all if you feel confident and secure and prepared for the problems you might face, then you will be able to tolerate the questions, doubts, and criticisms of others without feeling miserable or getting derailed.

How can I talk to my daycare provider about toilet training?

This can be a tricky relationship to begin with, as anyone who has ever faced it knows. Often this person insists that she "knows best," and her years of experience put her light-years beyond you in any matters involving childcare. The only response is that it is still your child, and you need to be able to communicate your desires for his care and have them respected. Try to explain why it is important, describe what you are doing at home, and keep your expectations clear. Make sure you know how she plans to handle accidents. Ideally, set up a schedule so that the sitter is putting the baby on the potty at about the same times that you do.

Many of you will find that your caregiver, especially if she is from another country, prefers to get your child out of diapers and is relieved that you are doing it in a way that is more traditionally familiar to her. In the end it has been well established that children in daycare environments are healthier and that everyone (including the provider) gets fewer gastrointestinal illnesses if the children are toilet trained. If she knows these facts, then it should be one of her goals to get all of the toddlers in her care out of diapers as soon as possible. Keep the lines of communication open, be receptive to her concerns and input, and make a plan that works for everyone. At the very least you should be able to start bringing your child in cloth pants with a waterproof cover, and that can be the first step to helping him and converting your caregiver to your plan.

What do you think about disposable diapers?

My husband once commented (when we were talking about potty training) that if convenience was a strong enough excuse to put someone in diapers, then he was getting a box for me before our next road trip. Obviously he was joking, but it really illustrates how terrible it is to leave children in diapers because we don't want to be inconvenienced. Can you imagine asking your seven-year-old to wear a diaper because you have a lot of errands to run and you don't want to take him to the potty? But asking this of a three-year-old seems perfectly okay, despite all of the medical evidence that she is just as likely to be able to use the potty.

Even at my house, we catch one another putting the baby in diapers and explain why it was necessary because of special circumstances. It is a running joke, actually, among my husband, my nanny, and me about who is the worst offender. Once we rushed out of the door to get pizza with the kids after work, and in the middle of dinner, I got a sinking feeling and asked my husband if he knew what our thirteen-month-old daughter was wearing under her clothes. He said he didn't know, and we both looked over at our adorable, babbling daughter in the high chair as though she had just become a potential enemy combatant. I didn't have anything with me, and if her clothes got all wet, then we were (all) totally out of luck. After an encouraging, knowing look from Dad, I went over to check out the situation (training pants, with waterproof pants on over, in case you were interested). We made a mental note to buy gifts for the nanny whenever possible. Those are funny parental moments, in retrospect, but I admit at the time I felt that the whole enterprise was insane.

More important, children in disposable diapers do not develop the concept that they must have frequent interruptions in their activities to be changed or to go potty. With some of the most modern materials used in disposable diapers, I often have parents tell me that they have to change their toddler only two or three times a day. This is very different from what nature (and independence from diapers) demands in terms of attention to potty habits. Is it really surprising that so many three-year-old children have decided that they prefer the convenience of diapers to the demands of using the potty? If adults find it too inconvenient and frustrating to frequently take a child to the potty and hate to interrupt their (incredibly busy) routines to get their child quickly to the toilet and take off his clothes so many times a day, then how must the child feel? His days are equally full; the work that he does is equally important and engaging to him. We are supposed to teach him to anticipate the need to go potty, to plan for it (and around it), to tolerate interruptions in his play to go potty, and to have the patience for an occasional accident.

There are some definite benefits to disposable diapers in terms of preventing diaper rashes. With the ultra-absorbent materials used today, many babies never get a diaper rash no matter how infrequently they are changed. They are also very convenient, and there are certain situations in which they can make a significant difference in your life. Use them when they are necessary, but as your baby gets older you should treat them almost like a guilty pleasure. They make your life easier in the short term, but prolonged use undercuts many things your child is striving to accomplish.

How do you handle rashes in the diaper area?

The problem of diaper rash becomes much more significant when you switch over to cotton pants. Disposable diapers pull the moisture away from your baby's skin. This is bad for helping her learn about toilet training, but it does protect her from rashes. The first solution is to change her more frequently. Most rashes are a reminder that someone didn't change her quickly enough, and some kids can't tolerate sitting in any wetness at all. It helps if you can (logistically) dress her in cotton pants without any cover, because it is obvious immediately when she goes potty, and you can get her cleaned up right away. It also helps to have some time with a bare bottom, so if your situation allows for that, then I encourage it.

Once your child has a rash, it is best to expose it to the air as much as possible. When putting her in pants, use a zinc oxide–based diaper cream (generic plain old zinc oxide is just fine) to help those areas heal. If the rash is worsening, or is starting to look like a lot of red dots spreading away from the central rash, then you can try some topical anti-fungal cream on the external areas of the rash. If things are not getting better, then it is time to visit your doctor.

What about the environmental impact of diapers?

The environmental impact of diapers is a topic that concerns a lot of parents. This issue has been studied by multiple people and most agree on the final analysis. Joyce Smith and Norma Pitts published a Fact Sheet from Ohio State University that referred to the published data from the EPA and others, and summarizes the various environmental effects of both types of diapers (available online at http://www.mindfully.org).

The report states that the average child uses over 5,000 diapers if he is toilet trained before 30 months of age. This results in 16 billion diapers or 2.7 million tons of disposable diapers requiring disposal every year. Nearly $300 million is spent annually to discard disposables. There are ongoing questions about the decomposition of both chemical and plastic parts of disposable diapers in landfills, and more than 250,000 trees are consumed each year to produce the wood pulp that provides the materials for disposable diapers. Furthermore, there are ongoing concerns that viral and bacterial material in soiled diapers might seep from landfills and enter ground water supplies, though to date, no evidence of diaper waste causing disease in community water systems has been identified.

By comparison, cotton used to manufacture cloth diapers is often treated with pesticides, and requires water and energy resources to cultivate and transport. Laundering of cloth diapers utilizes water and energy resources, and chemical products are used to clean them that contribute to water pollution and also tax municipal water treatment systems. A 1990 study showed that cloth diapers used twice as much energy and four times as much water as disposables, and created greater air and water pollution than disposables. Commerical diaper services increase these problems because they add fuel use and air pollution from delivery trucks. There are organic cotton diapers and training pants available (made from cotton grown without the use of pesticides), and more environmentally friendly detergents that can be used to clean diapers.

Unless you live in area with specific environmental concerns such as particularly limited water supply or extremely over-burdened landfills, the environmental impact of disposables versus cloth diapers is closely balanced. The important issue to consider in all of this is how long the child is in diapers, and that the best thing for the environment is to get him out of diapers sooner rather than later. An extra six months or year in diapers adds up to a lot of waste and pollution, either way. There is ample evidence that the earlier children are exposed to their own body's signals (and that means getting them into cloth pants), the sooner they will be trained. I think that the environmental advantage of earlier potty training makes doing so extra worth it.

My daughter was completely trained at eighteen months, but my son is two and a half and still has frequent accidents. Is that normal?

Every study about potty training that made an effort to separate boys and girls in the results has confirmed that girls (in general) are trained earlier than boys. The reason for this is not known. The reality is that the variability among all children with regard to when they will reliably be trained is much greater than the difference between boys and girls. So I would focus much more on the fact that they are simply two different individuals, rather than on the idea that he is taking longer because he is a boy.

The number of accidents an individual child has is related to his body (including his brain and many inborn traits), as well as to his personality. Many people notice that their more active children have more frequent accidents, simply because it is hard for them to take those breaks to go potty. I have observed that many highly intelligent kids have frequent accidents because they are concentrating so intently on the work that they are doing that they forget to take a break. In the end it is a highly variable thing, and you must remember that both of these children are normal. You may need to make certain modifications with your approach to each of your children, such as monitoring fluid intake more closely or giving more frequent reminders, but that is all considered normal in the scheme of things.

My child hates to sit on the potty. What do I do?

It depends on the age of the child. If you are starting at a young age, and you are seeing this type of reaction in a baby, just be patient and keep trying. In most cases, it is a stage that passes very quickly. Continue to sit her on the potty in a routine way, and if she protests, then do not force her. I think it really helps to incorporate the potty into diaper changes. So when you go to change a diaper, sit the baby on the potty before you put a new one on. The stage will pass, just as temporary resistance to her crib, high chair, car seat, or stroller usually does. Make sure it is a pleasant experience and that you are giving her your full attention for those few moments on the potty. Most small children are happy doing anything if it involves getting someone's undivided attention, and a board book or a toy is an appropriate transitional object if she is anxious.

For older children it depends on when you started. If you have an older child whom you are starting to train for the first time, and she is resistant, then refer to Chapter 4. If you have a child who was cooperating with training for a period of time and suddenly does not want to, then one of two things is happening. The first and most important one to realize is that something like a hard stool or a urinary tract infection might be making her uncomfortable. Vaginitis in little girls does the same thing. So it is not a bad idea to check with your doctor if toilet refusal occurs all of a sudden.

The second cause is that your child is testing you or engaging in what we call a power struggle. You should take some time to think about your tactics. Are you putting too much pressure on her to go potty too frequently? Are you asserting too much control over her? Make sure that your techniques are appropriate for your child's age and maturity level. Maybe she needs a little more independence. Maybe she has had a few accidents and has gotten frustrated, and you should supervise her a little more closely. Sudden resistance to the potty or any increase in number of accidents is a good reason to take a look at everything that is going on with your child and to seek help from your doctor, a psychologist, or a therapist if you don't know what to do.

What do I do with my child who refuses to use a public washroom?

You are not alone. I have had so many parents ask the same question. The first (and most obvious) thing is to try to avoid the situation. Make sure that everyone goes potty on the way out the door and that you plan ahead. There are a couple of tricks when the situation is unavoidable. First, buy a little fold-up seat cover to carry in your diaper bag. You can get these from many baby stores, and they make your child feel so much more secure on a big potty. You can try to let him stand on the seat and go (this only works for urine). In the most extreme case put an extra potty in the trunk of your car, and go out to use it if he flatly refuses the public washrooms. Of course there are some situations in which none of these things will be possible, and that is just part of growing up. Try to be calm yourself, and don't let him see how stressed-out public washrooms make you. Make sure he washes his hands well, but don't give him a lecture about germs and diseases that leaves him terrified.

How should I talk to my child about accidents?

In many ways that is the wrong question to ask. It should be "How should I *handle* accidents?" because the way that you respond to these situations will determine how your child feels much more than what you tell her. When your child is small (under eighteen months of age), you just get her changed into dry pants without a fuss. Ideally you do this in the bathroom, and you can talk to her with phrases like "You went potty" to start to teach her the vocabulary and build an association. If possible I often sit her on the potty before I put her dry pants on because it really reinforces that association, and you will be surprised how often she stops going when she feels the wetness and will finish going on the potty.

As your child gets older she may get upset or even throw a tantrum when she has an accident. You should stay as calm as possible (and this can be hard when there is furniture—especially other people's furniture—involved). Let your child know that everything is fine, nobody is mad at her, and she needs to get some clean pants on. You can say things like "We forgot to get to the potty because we were so busy playing." Try to avoid any recrimination or questions like "*Why* did you have an accident?" That question sounds ridiculous to a child who certainly did not mean to or want to have an accident.

If she does want to talk to you about it, then let her know that accidents are a normal part of learning about the potty and that all children have them sometimes. Sometimes it helps to use a specific example like "Even your cousin Johnny had accidents sometimes when he was your age, but now he goes on the potty every time." Let her know that you love her lots, and that you will try to help her to re-member to go potty before she has an emergency next time. Most important, be prepared. Getting her dry and back to play without much fuss is going to reassure her more than anything else.

How should I handle bed-wetting?

When your child awakens in the middle of the night complaining that he is wet, there are a few options open to you, and what you should do depends a lot on your child's age and personality. Often the wetness woke him up and he stopped going before his bladder was empty, so he should go to the washroom and sit on the potty. This should not be like a punishment, but you should tell him to try to go potty before he puts on dry pajamas. You can let him crawl into bed with you and deal with his sheets in the morning, or you can pull off the wet sheets and fix his bed for him right then. I admit there were times when my kids were small that I would hear a little voice next to my bed saying "Mommy, I am wet," and I would just pull off his wet clothes and pull him into bed with me. This led to a period of time with my first child in which he started to prefer to sleep naked and demanded to have his pajamas off before he would go to bed every night. My husband did *not* appreciate the naked four-year-old running around the house every morning, so I tried to limit this tactic. My sec-ond child would never go for it anyway and demanded that I go and get him pajamas before he would go back to sleep. As far as I am concerned you do whatever works between the hours of midnight and five in the morning.

Older children may prefer to have clean sheets available

to them so that they can deal with the whole thing themselves. At what age they can handle a wet bed without help varies from child to child. Some can do it when they are four, especially if you make it easy for them. Some seven-year-olds will need your help. A lot of it depends on how frequently bed-wetting occurs. There are many waterproof pads available, either as a whole mattress pad or as just a smaller pad (like those used in hospitals) that goes under the sheet in the area on which your child's bottom lies. If he has frequent accidents, then all you need is some extra pads and a flat sheet and the child can get things at least workable until the morning.

Remember that bed-wetting is really common in kids under seven years of age, and there is no room for punishment of any kind. It is totally appropriate to think about what you did the night before and how much he had to drink after dinner. Talking to him about these habits can help him feel in control of the situation, as well. Often it is obvious that he was overtired from extra activity the day before or had an extra treat or drink before bed. In those situations you just reinforce good behaviors and don't make a big deal out of it. If it happens frequently, then you need to set specific limits on his evening fluids and make sure he tries to go potty immediately before bed (even if he just went). If he still has frequent accidents, then you may want to wake him when you are going to bed to empty his bladder again. By doing things like this for short periods of time you can often break the habit. Otherwise there are alarms and other training devices available through your doctor or pharmacy that can help a lot, as well as very effective medications for older children.

How did you potty train your own kids?

This is probably the most frequent question I hear. I have provided the answer throughout this book, but my direct answer is also helpful. First of all I used disposable diapers on all of my kids in the first year of life. This was mostly for convenience but also because they almost never got rashes if I changed them frequently enough. Parents who use cloth from the beginning have my respect and admiration, but in the end I am a practical girl.

My first son started sitting on the potty once a day when he was about nine months of age. He was cared for at home, and we started sitting him on the potty after breakfast. He was a pretty easygoing and complacent baby, and he was happy to sit there from the beginning. We put him there and then sat right in front of him with a board book (which he loved) and read it to him. He was so content with the whole thing; he never tried to get up and was happy as long as you were talking to him. He usually had a bowel movement at this time and in fact never had a messy diaper again.

We gradually increased the number of times he sat on the potty, adding a time after nap, after dinner, before bath, before bed, and when he woke up in the morning. We followed the same routine, just had him sit and look at a board book and then get up after a minute or two. He started wearing cotton training pants when he was about fifteen months old, and I totally eliminated diapers when he was eighteen months old. He was dry at night pretty much from that point, and had a few bed-wetting accidents over the years, usually when he was overtired. He started preschool at three years of age and had a few wetting accidents as he transitioned to the new environment, but that passed quickly.

My second son was a little quicker to lunge forward when we started to sit him on the potty at about seven months of age. He was an active baby who always wanted to escape and explore. We did the same thing in terms of introducing the potty, but he would often lean forward and try to crawl away or stand up. We would get his pants back on and try again later when this happened. He hit a point after a year of age when he started having his bowel movements on the toilet, and he was so happy with that that he was much more patient to sit. We got rid of the diapers at about fifteen months of age, and he had one or two accidents a day unless I was really taking him to the potty frequently. This lasted until he was about twenty months of age, when the accidents drastically decreased, he became regularly dry at night, and things started to fall into place.

He still had more frequent accidents when he was busy playing or overtired than I had experienced with my first son, but he was reliably dry before he turned two. He wet his bed at times (usually it would happen every night for three or four nights and then not again for months), but this passed after he turned three. When he started preschool he had accidents about once a week for the first few months, but then that let up and he did well on his own.

My daughter was the one who would leap off the potty like a spring whenever we put her on it. In fact it was really a game to her from the time she was nine months old to laugh hysterically and lunge off the potty and crawl away as fast as possible. I found this very discouraging at the time, but by thirteen months of age she was willing to sit for a board book and then we started to fall into the usual training routine. She is into cotton training pants and really catching on at fifteen months of age. She is the one who gets really excited and proud of herself when she actually goes on the potty, and we really must cheer and clap for her every time. Actually she is perfectly happy to cheer and clap for herself, but that is another story entirely. The next edition of this book will have to tell the story of how she did in the preschool years. For now she wakes up dry and uses the potty, will usually sit after meals and after her nap, and frequently tells us when she needs to go potty.

epilogue

This energy of love is given us so that each shall have it in himself. Although the amount given to man is limited and diffused, it is the greatest of all the forces at his disposal. That part of it which we possess consciously is renewed every time a baby is born and, even if circumstances at a later stage cause it to become dormant, we still feel for it a fervent desire.

—Maria Montessori, THE ABSORBENT MIND

There is a growing buzz in the media about the increasing problems teenagers and young adults are having making the transition to independent adult life. It is commonly discussed by CEOs of large corporations that this generation of young workers coming out of college contains the brightest and most educated in history but they lack any sense of direction, any desire to achieve or contribute, and in many cases any sense of purpose or direction. I heard an interview with the great learning expert Dr. Mel Levine recently, in which he remarked that the complete inability to delay gratification, to work for a long period of time toward a goal, or to really plan for the future at all is so pervasive among young adults in our society that it is really considered normal.

Those of us who work in pediatrics see some of the earliest symptoms of this in our office daily. Almost every day I ask a sixteen- or seventeen-year-old about his plans for the future, and I have to try to decipher a mumbled "college . . . or whatever . . ." because he doesn't even look up at me. Many are so totally preoccupied with sports or other activities that their parents became nothing more than full-time recreation coordinators years ago. Most of the parents are too frightened by what they hear in the media (and often by what they have seen with others) to confront or place expectations on their children in any way. Parents have even told me "As long as he is not doing drugs and his grades are okay, I let him do whatever he wants."

A lot of the reasons for this have been discussed at length in the media. Our whole society practices the instant gratification lifestyle. Parents feel guilty because they feel that they can't give their kids as much as others, they aren't there enough, they are divorced, or they travel for work. They don't want their kids to hate them, and they have been bombarded with the idea that putting pressure on their kids will lead to rebellion. Somehow we have collectively come to the conclusion that placing demands and expectations on our children leads to insecurity, and that first and foremost children must feel accepted for who they are.

Those principles of acceptance and unconditional love are the essential underpinnings of family relationships, but obviously they do not translate literally into telling your child to do whatever he wants whenever he wants. So there is a line there (somewhere) where parents are supposed to step in and teach their kids that putting off something fun so that they can complete their work or meet a responsibility is part of life. Respecting others and honoring commitments are necessary parts of finding a place in the world. Making goals, accepting challenges, and dealing with both delayed gratification and occasional failure are essential skills for attaining success and making a contribution. Being resilient, resourceful, and responsive to your environment are essential parts of being successful and happy as an adult. As a society we are not teaching our kids these things, and the real responsibility is with parents.

What does this have to do with potty training? I hear some of the first indications of this philosophy when I talk about potty training with parents. Parents are afraid to place expectations on or even to set a schedule for their toddlers. They talk a lot about wanting their children to feel secure and accepted and very little about what their role is in teaching them skills that lead to independence, mastery, and confidence. They fear the effects of failure and setbacks on the children they so want to protect.

There was a family that I knew from my practice that had a daughter prematurely, and the baby spent several months in the NICU. She ended up having a rough first year of life, with very slow growth and weight gain, but then she really started to catch up and blossom and turned into a beautiful, totally normal little girl. I brought up potty training with her parents at the fifteen-month visit, and the mom said "This little girl doesn't have to be potty trained until she is ten years old if she doesn't want to." And I just thought, Wow, that is the problem right there. I totally understood where her sentiment was coming from, all of those feelings of guilt and the desire to protect her baby. But her response was all wrong. She should have asked "What can I do to help her succeed, how can I teach her and help her, and what should I expect from her?"

The fact is that children are naturally resilient. They fall down and get right up. They taste new foods and spit them out if they dislike them, happy to go on eating the next thing available. They walk up to strangers and then scamper away when they feel that they have overstepped their confidence. We must not be the ones discouraging them from trying, holding them back, and causing their expectations of the world to be completely wrong. From the time that they are small we can show them that people who love them have expectations for them. They should feel that those expectations are flexible but fundamentally unchanging. They should learn about planning, about putting off enjoyable activities to attend to other demands or responsibilities, and about the importance of personal goals from very early in childhood.

I firmly believe that children are not afraid of failure, but we instill that in them by being overly protective and showing them how distressing it is to us (the people who love them) to see them struggle. We must allow them to find their way and then provide the structure, advice, and example of how to succeed. Then whatever kind of success they find in life will be recognized and appreciated. Most of all they will learn to face a challenge or a failure by looking at themselves for both solutions and strength. They will know that real happiness and success take work and that security and self-confidence develop out of their own abilities, work, and mastery. And then they will apply those ideals throughout their lives. At least that's what I hope for my kids, and I try to remember it as an ideal when I find myself loving them so much that I am getting in their way.

resources

Cotton Training Pants

I look for soft cotton products, but those with polyester side panels to add stretch for a better fit are also fine. Most training pants have some added layers of fabric in the center to absorb a small amount of fluid so that accidents are more contained. They should be affordable, so you don't worry too much if you need to discard a pair in an awkward situation. And they should be comfortable and easy for your child to pull up and down.

- **Gerber**'s training pants are inexpensive, soft, and long-lasting. A staple! Available at Target, www.gerberchildrenswear.com, or www.clothdiaper.com.

- **Hanna Andersson**'s pants are more expensive, but are soft and durable, like little luxury training pants. Available at www.hannaandersson.com.

- **Under the Nile** makes a 100% organic cotton training pant that is very nice. Available at www.underthenile.com or www.inourforrest.com.

Waterproof Covers

I look for vinyl products because they are softer and more comfortable, and less likely to crack with washing. They should pull on easily so the child can feel independent. Remember, the waterproof covers will not absorb all the liquid, so all will eventually leak. This is part of the plan; children are not supposed to sit in the same wet pants for hours!

- **Dappi,** available at www.babybestbuy.com or www.cottonbabies.com.

- **Gerber** vinyl covers, available at www.gerberchildrenswear.com.

Potty

In my opinion Baby Bjorn makes one of the best potty chairs out there. It comes in two sturdy pieces, is just the right height, provides some back support, is easy to clean, and is affordable. There are countless potty options, but in general avoid potty chairs that have a lot of pieces, might feel unstable to the child, or can't be fully cleaned. **Baby Bjorn** is available at Babies "R" Us or www.babybjorn.com.

Children's Books

These classic picture books can be helpful and entertaining when teaching your baby how to use the potty.

- *I Have to Go* (Sesame Street Toddler Books) by Anna Ross (Random House Books for Young Readers)

- *Everyone Poops* by Taro Gomi (Kane/Miller Book Publishers)

- *Once Upon a Potty (Girl)* and *Once Upon a Potty (Boy)* by Alona Frankel (HarperFestival)

Interested in Infant Potty Training?

Two websites with resources, links, and information are www.diaperfreebaby.org and www.white-boucke.com.

bibliography

American Academy of Pediatrics. Task Force on Circumcision. "Circumcision policy statement." *Pediatrics*, 103 (3) (1999) 686–693.

Ariès, Philippe. *Centuries of Childhood: A Social History of Family Life*. New York: Alfred A. Knopf, Inc., 1962.

Azrin, Nathan H., and Richard M. Foxx. *Toilet Training Persons with Developmental Disabilities*. Champaign, IL: Research Press, 1973.

———. *Toilet Training in Less Than a Day*. New York: Pocket Books, 1974.

Bakker, Els, et al. "Results of a questionnaire evaluating the effects of different methods of toilet training on achieving bladder control." *BJU International* 90 (2002) 456–461.

Bakker, Els, and J. van Gool and Jean-Jacques Wyndaele. "Results of a questionnaire evaluating different aspects of personal and familial situation, and the methods of potty-training in two groups of children with a different outcome of bladder control." *Scandinavian Journal of Urology and Nephrology*, 35 (2001) 370–376.

Bakker, Els, and Jean-Jacques Wyndaele. "Changes in the toilet training of children during the last 60 years: The cause of an increase in lower urinary tract dysfunction?" *BJU International*, 86 (2000) 248–252.

Bakwin, Harry. "Enuresis in children." *Journal of Pediatrics*, 58 (6) (1961) 806–819.

Berk, Lawrence B., and Patrick C. Friman. "Epidemiologic aspects of toilet training." *Clinical Pediatrics*, 29 (5) (1990) 278–282.

Blum, Nathan J., and B. Taubman and M. L. Osborne. "Behavioral characteristics of children with stool toileting refusal." *Journal of Pediatrics*, 99 (1) (1997) 50–53.

Borowitz, Stephen M., et al. "Treatment of childhood encopresis: A randomized trial comparing three treatment protocols." *Journal of Pediatric Gastroenterology and Nutrition*, 34 (2002) 378–384.

Brayden, Robert M., and Stephen R. Poole. "Common behavioral problems in infants and children." *Primary Care*, 22 (1) (1995) 81–97.

Brazelton, T. B. "A child-oriented approach to toilet training." *Pediatrics*, 29 (1962) 121–128.

Brazelton, T. B., et al. "Instruction, timeliness, and medical influences affecting toilet training." *Pediatrics*, 103 (6) (1999) 1353–1358.

Brooks, Robert C., et al. "Review of the treatment literature for encopresis, functional constipation, and stool-toileting refusal." *Annals of Behavioral Medicine*, 22 (3) (2000) 260–267.

Carlson, Susan, and Russell Asnes. "Maternal expectations and attitudes toward toilet training: A comparison between clinic mothers and private practice mothers." *Journal of Pediatrics*, 84 (1) (1974) 148–151.

Chamberlin, Robert W., Jr. "Approaches to child rearing—Their identification and classification." *Clinical Pediatrics*, 4 (3) (1965) 150–159.

Christophersen, Edward R. "Toilet problems in children." *Pediatric Annals*, 20 (1991) 240–244.

Cicero, Frank R., and Al Pfadt. "Investigation of a reinforcement-based toilet training procedure for children with autism." *Research in Developmental Disabilities*, 23 (2002) 319–331.

Craig, Jonathan C., et al. "Effect of circumcision on incidence of urinary tract infection in preschool boys." *Journal of Pediatrics*, 128 (1) (1996) 23–27.

DeVries, Marten W., and M. Rachel deVries. "Cultural relativity of toilet training readiness: A perspective from East Africa." *Pediatrics*, 60 (2) (1977) 170–177.

Fishman, Laurie, et al. "Early constipation and toilet training in children with encopresis." *Journal of Pediatric Gastroenterology and Nutrition*, 34 (2002) 385–388.

Ford, Frank R. *Diseases of the Central Nervous System in Infancy, Childhood and Adolescence*. Springfield, IL: Charles C. Thomas Publisher, 1952.

Friman, Patrick C. "A preventative context for enuresis." *Pediatric Clinics of North America*, 33 (4) (1986) 871–886.

Gerrard, Sterling D., and Julius B. Richmond. "Psychogenic megacolon manifested by fecal soiling." *Pediatrics*, 10 (1952) 474–483.

Gesell, Arnold. *Developmental Schedules*. New York: The Psychological Corporation, 1949.

Gesell, Arnold, and Catherine Strunk Amatruda. *Developmental Diagnosis: Normal and Abnormal Child Development*. New York: Harper and Row, 1941.

Glicklich, Lucille B. "An historical account of enuresis." *Pediatrics*, 8 (1951) 859–875.

Goellner, Mark H., and E. E. Ziegler and S. J. Fomon. "Urination during the first three years of life." *Nephron*, 28 (1981) 174–178.

Hadler, Stephen C., et al. "Risk factors for hepatitis A in day-care centers." *Journal of Infectious Diseases*, 145 (2) (1982) 255–261.

Hadler, Steven C., and Louise L. McFarland. "Hepatitis in day care centers: Epidemiology and prevention." *Review of Infectious Diseases*, 8 (4) (1986) 548–557.

Hellström, Anna-Lena. "Influence of potty training habits on dysfunctional bladder in children." *Lancet*, 356 (2000) 1787.

Hindley, C. B. "Growing up in five countries: A comparison of data on weaning, elimination training, age of walking and IQ in relation to social class from European longitudinal studies." *Developmental Medicine and Child Neurology*, 10 (1968) 715–724.

Holmdahl, Gundela, et al. "Four-hour voiding observation in healthy infants." *Journal of Urology*, 156 (1996) 1809–1812.

Howe, Allison C., and C. Eugene Walker. "Behavioral management of toilet training, enuresis, and encopresis." *Pediatric Clinics of North America*, 39 (3) (1992) 413–432.

Huschka, Mabel. "The child's response to coercive bowel training." *Psychosomatic Medicine*, 2 (1950) 301–308.

Hutch, John A., and Charles E. Shopfner. "The lateral cystogram as an aid to urologic diagnosis." *Journal of Urology*, 99 (1968) 292–296.

Issenman, Robert M., and Robert B. Filmer and Peter A. Gorski. "A review of bowel and bladder control development in children: How gastrointestinal and urologic conditions relate to problems in toilet training." *Pediatrics*, 103 (6) (1999) 1346–1352.

Jansson, U.-B., et al. "Voiding pattern in healthy children 0 to 3 years old: A longitudinal study." *Journal of Urology*, 164 (2000) 2050–2054.

Kinservik, Margo A., and Margaret M. Friedhoff. "Control issues in toilet training." *Pediatric Nursing*, 26 (3) (2000) 267–272.

Klackenberg, G. "A prospective longitudinal study of children: Data on psychic health and development up to 8 years of age." *Acta Paediatrica Scandinavica Supplementum*, 224 (1971) 1–239.

Largo, Remo H., et al. "Development of bladder and bowel control: Significance of prematurity, perinatal risk factors, psychomotor development and gender." *European Journal of Pediatrics*, 158 (1999) 115–122.

———. "Does a profound change in toilet training affect development of bowl and bladder control?" *Developmental Medicine and Child Neurology*, 38 (1996) 1106–1116.

Largo, Remo H., and Werner Stutzle. "Longitudinal study of bowel and bladder control by day and at night in the first six years of life. I: Epidemiology and interrelations between bowel and bladder control." *Developmental Medicine and Child Neurology*, 19 (1977) 598–606.

———. "Longitudinal study of bowel and bladder control by day and at night in the first six years of life. II: The role of potty-training and the child's initiative." *Developmental Medicine and Child Neurology*, 19 (1977) 607–613.

Leiderman, P. H., et al. "African infant precocity and some social influences during the first year." *Nature* (1973) 242:249.

Levine, Melvin D. "Children with encopresis: A descriptive analysis." *Pediatrics*, 56 (3) (1975) 412–416.

Levine, Melvin D., and Harry Bakow. "Children with encopresis: A study of treatment outcome." *Journal of Pediatrics*, 58 (1976) 845–852.

Luxem, Michael, and Edward Christophersen. "Behavioral toilet training in early childhood: Research, practice and implications." *Journal of Developmental and Behavioral Pediatrics*, 15 (1994) 370–378.

MacKeith, Ronald C., and S. R. Meadow and R. K. Turner. "How children become dry." *Clinics in Developmental Medicine*, 49 (1973) 3–32.

Martin, John A., et al. "Secular trends and individual differences in toilet-training progress." *Journal of Pediatric Psychology*, 9 (4) (1984) 457–467.

McGraw, M. B. "Neural maturation as exemplified in achievement of bladder control." *Journal of Pediatrics* (1940) 580–590.

Michel, Robert S. "Toilet training." *Pediatrics in Review*, 20 (7) (1999) 240–244.

Monsen, Rita B. "Giving children control and toilet training." *Journal of Pediatric Nursing*, 16 (5) (2001) 375–376.

Montessori, Maria. *The Absorbent Mind*. New York: Henry Holt and Company, 1995.

Muellner, S. R. "Development of urinary control in children." *Journal of the American Medical Association*, 172 (1960) 1256–1261.

Oppel, Wallace C., and Paul A. Harper and Rowland V. Rider. "The age of attaining bladder control." *Pediatrics*, 42 (4) (1968) 614–624.

Orlansky, Harold. "Infant Care and Personality." *Psychology Bulletin*, 46 (1949) 1–48.

Pickering, Larry K., and Alfred V. Bartlett and W. E. Woodward. "Acute infectious diarrhea among children in day care: Epidemiology and control." *Review of Infectious Diseases*, 8 (4) (1986) 539–547.

Pinkerton, Philip. "Psychogenic megacolon in children: The implications of bowel negativism." *Archives of Diseases in Childhood*, 33 (1958) 371–380.

Rappaport, Leonard A., and Melvin D. Levine. "The prevention of constipation and encopresis: A developmental model and approach." *Pediatric Clinics of North America*, 33 (4) (1986) 859–869.

Roberts, Katherine E., and Judith A. Schoellkopf. "Eating, sleeping, and elimination practices of a group of two-and-one-half-year-old children." *American Journal of Diseases in Children*, 82 (1951) 137–143.

Robson, William L., and Alexander K. Leung. "Advising parents on toilet training." *American Family Physician*, 44 (1991) 1263–1266.

Rogers, June. "Cognitive bladder training in the community." *Paediatric Nursing*, 8 (8) (1996) 18–20.

Rubin, Greg. "Constipation." *Clinical Evidence*, 7 (2002) 292–296.

Schmitt, Barton D. "Toilet training refusal: Avoid the battle and win the war." *Contemporary Pediatrics*, Dec. (1987) 32–50.

Schum, Timothy R., et al. "Factors associated with toilet training in the 1990s." *Ambulatory Pediatrics*, 1 (2) (2001) 79–86.

———. "Sequential acquisition of toilet-training skills: A descriptive study of gender and age differences in normal children (Abstract)." *Pediatrics*, 109 (3) (2002).

Sears, Robert R., and Eleanor E. Maccoby and Harry T. Levin. "Toilet training." In *Patterns of Child Rearing*, edited by Robert R. Sears, Eleanor E. Maccoby, and Harry T. Levin, 102–137. Evanston, IL: Row, Peterson and Company, 1957.

Sillén, Ulla, et al. "Control of voiding means better emptying of the bladder in children with congenital dilating VUR." *BJU International*, 85 (Suppl. 4) (2000) 13.

Singh-Grewal, D., and J. Macdessi and J. Craig. "Circumcision for the prevention of urinary tract infection in boys: A systematic review of randomized trials and observational studies." *Archives of Diseases in Childhood*, 90 (8) (2005) 853–858.

Smeets, Paul M., et al. "Shaping self-initiated toileting in infants." *Journal of Applied Behavior Analysis*, 18 (1985) 303–308.

Smith, Joyce A. and Norma Pitts. "The Diaper Delusion: Not a Clear Issue." http://www.mindfully.org/Plastic/Diaper-Not-Clear.htm.

Spock, Benjamin. *The Common Sense Book of Baby and Child Care*. New York: Dual Sloan and Pierce, 1946.

———. *Baby and Child Care*. New York: Pocket Books, 1957.

Stadtler, Ann C., and Peter A. Gorski and T. B. Brazelton. "Toilet training methods, clinical interventions, and recommendations." *Pediatrics* 103 (6) (1999) 1359–1361.

Stadtler, Ann C. "Preventing encopresis." *Pediatric Nursing*, 15 (3) (1989) 282–284.

Stehbens, James A., and David L. Silber. "Parental expectations in toilet training." *Pediatrics*, 48 (1971) 451–454.

Stendler, Celia B. "Sixty years of child training practices: Revolution in the nursery." *Journal of Pediatrics*, 36 (1950) 122.

Stephens, J. A., and David L. Silber. "Parental expectations vs. outcome in toilet training." *Pediatrics*, 54 (4) (1974) 493–495.

Sullivan, Peggy, et al. "Longitudinal study of occurrence of diarrheal disease in day care centers." *American Journal of Public Health*, 74 (9) (1984) 987–991.

Sweet, Clifford. "Enuresis, psychologic problems of childhood." *Journal of the American Medical Association*, 132 (1946) 279–281.

Takahashi, E. "Investigation of the age release from the diaper environment." *Pediatrician*, 14 (1987) 48–52.

Taubman, Bruce. "Toilet training and toileting refusal for stool only: A prospective study." *Pediatrics*, 99 (1) (1997) 54–58.

Taubman, Bruce, and Marianne Buzby. "Overflow encopresis and stool toileting refusal during toilet training: A prospective study on the effect of therapeutic efficacy." *Journal of Pediatrics* (1997) 768–771.

To, Teresa, et al. "Cohort study on circumcision of newborn boys and subsequent risk of urinary-tract infection." *Lancet*, 352 (9143) (1998) 1813–1816.

Van der Plas, Roos N., et al. "Treatment of defecation problems in children: The role of education, demystification and toilet training." *European Journal of Pediatrics*, 156 (1997) 689–692.

Vincent, C. E. "Trends in infant care ideas." *Child Development*, 22 (1951) 199–209.

Warren, N., and J. M. Parkin. "A neurological and behavioral comparison of African and European newborns in Uganda." *Child Development*, 45 (4) (1974) 966–971.

Weir, Kirk. "Night and day wetting among a population of three-year-olds." *Developmental Medicine and Child Neurology*, 24 (1982) 479–484.

Whiting, John W. M., and Irving L. Child. *Child Training and Personality*. New Haven: Yale University Press, 1953.

Wiener, John S., et al. "Long-term efficacy of simple behavioral therapy for daytime wetting in children." *Journal of Urology*, 164 (2000) 786–790.

Wiswell, Thomas E., and Dietrich W. Geschke. "Risks from circumcision during the first month of life compared with those for uncircumcised boys." *Pediatrics*, 83 (6) (1989) 1011–1015.

Wolfenstein, Martha. "Trends in infant care." *American Journal of Orthopsychiatry*, 23 (1953) 120–130.

Yeung, C. K., et al. "Natural filling cystometry in infants and children." *British Journal of Urology*, 75 (1995) 531–537.

Yeung, C. K., et al. "Some new insights into bladder function in infancy." *British Journal of Urology*, 76 (1995) 235–240.

Young, G. C. "The relationship of 'potting' to enuresis." *Journal of the Royal Institute of Public Health*, 27 (1964) 23–24.

index

about the author

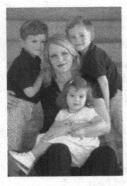

Jill Lekovic, MD, FAAP, is a Board Certified Pediatrician and a member of the Faculty of the Department of Pediatrics at St. Joseph's Hospital and Medical Center in Phoenix, Arizona. She received a bachelor's degree from the University of Chicago with Honors and went on to earn a Doctor of Medicine degree from the University of Illinois at Chicago, where she was inducted into the Alpha Omega Alpha national medical honor society. Dr. Lekovic completed her residency training in Pediatrics at the University of Illinois at Chicago Hospitals. She lives in Phoenix with her husband Gregory and their three children.